PLANNING FOR THE NEEDS OF PEOPLE WITH DEMENTIA

Planning for the Needs of People with Dementia

The development of a profile for use in local services

DR P. SPICKER
Senior Lecturer in Social Policy, University of Dundee

DR D.S. GORDON
Research and Development Manager, Lanarkshire Health Board

With
Dr B. Ballinger
Consultant Psychiatrist, Royal Dundee Liff Hospital
Ms B. Gillies
Senior Lecturer in Social Work, University of Dundee
Mrs N. McWilliam
Care Manager, Dundee City Council
Dr W. Mutch
Unit Medical Manager, Medicine for the Elderly, Tayside Health Board
Dr P. Seed
Department of Social Work, University of Dundee

Avebury

Aldershot • Brookfield USA • Hong Kong • Singapore • Sydney

Published by
Avebury
Ashgate Publishing Limited
Gower House
Croft Road
Aldershot
Hants GU11 3HR
England

Ashgate Publishing Company
Old Post Road
Brookfield
Vermont 05036
USA

British Library Cataloguing in Publication Data
Spicker, Paul
Planning for the needs of people with dementia : the development of a profile for use in local services
1.Dementia - Patients - Services for 2.Medical care - Needs assessment 3.Health planning
I.Title II.Gordon, David S. III.Ballinger, B.
362.1'968983

Library of Congress Catalog Card Number: 96-79373

ISBN 1 85972 600 3

Printed in Great Britain by the Ipswich Book Company, Suffolk

Contents

List of tables

Acknowledgements

This book is based on work funded by the Scottish Office, grant no. K/OPR/2/2/C978. At the time of the project, Dr Gordon was Epidemiologist, Forth Valley Health Board; Brenda Gillies and Nancy McWilliam were Research Assistants in the Department of Medicine, University of Dundee. The project was located in the Department of Medicine, University of Dundee. Katie Horne worked as the project's secretary.

The project involved the co-operation of a large number of professionals and carers, without whose help the work would not have feasible. We also took the advice of a consultative group. This group comprised:

Health service

Dr K Adam, Consultant in Public Health Medicine, Tayside Health Board
Dr B Goudie, General Practitioner (until Dec. 1993)
Mrs H Jenkins, Director of Nursing Services, Perth
Mrs J Hays, Assistant Director, Community Nursing, Forfar (Angus)
Mr J Macleod, Director of Nursing and Quality Assurance, Royal Dundee Liff Hospital

Social work

Ms J Ridley, Tayside Social Work Department
Mrs L Douthwaite, Unit Manager, Occupational Therapy Services
Miss A Crawford, Group Manager (Community Care), Arbroath (Angus)
Mrs I Crichton, Senior Care Manager, Kirriemuir (Angus)
Mrs A Mill, Sheltered Housing Officer, Arbroath (Angus)

Other

Dr C Cohen, Consultant Geriatrician (retired)
Mrs I Anderson, Dundee Carers Group
Ms S Melvin, Training Officer, Northern College, Dundee.

Their support is gratefully acknowledged.

1 Introduction

This book describes the work of a three-year project funded by the Scottish Office to develop an instrument for use by local planners to assess the needs of people with dementia. At that level, it can be read as the report of a field project. The research was intended to serve planners working with dementia, mainly in health and social services. The work has thrown up some important information about people with dementia, which means that it will be of interest more widely to people with an interest in social gerontology, while the method and approach should be of interest to people planning for other dependent groups.

At the same time, the book considers a much wider range of issues concerned with the process of planning to meet needs, including:

- the problems of people with dementia
- problems in the measurement of need
- ways of identifying the population with dementia, and
- the process of planning services to meet needs.

Approach

The instrument which was devised for this project, the Tayside Profile for Dementia Planning, is not intended to be used for individual assessments, but rather to provide information about the total range of problems for which services are to be provided. It does this by constructing a profile of people's needs across a range of factors, including problems with mobility, problems with self-care and continence, need for domestic support, problems with behaviour, the social contacts of the person with dementia and the position of carers. This information can be used in several different ways by planners:

- to identify the needs for particular services

- to identify needs which are unmet, and
- to see what effect different kinds of services will have on the population which is being served.

The plan of the book

In chapters 2-4, the book lays out an approach to planning and the design of a profile as a means to compile information about needs. Chapters 5-9 describe the fieldwork for the project, which involved a service-based census of people with dementia, assessment of a sample of those censused, and processes to test the profile in practice. The information in these chapters is more specialised, but several issues raised in them are of general importance. In particular, the methods which are used both to identify the population and subsequently to assess their needs are, we believe, extendable to other settings and other kinds of dependent group. Chapter 10 shows how the information used in the profile might be applied. The discussion of ethical issues, in chapter 11, is a further consideration related to fieldwork, but it also relates to wider issues, and for that reason it has been treated separately from the main discussion of fieldwork. The final chapter briefly reviews the profile in the light of the criteria established at the outset of the book.

2 Dementia, needs and service planning

Needs

Needs as problems

'Needs' refer, in the first place, to the kinds of problem which people experience: people who suffer from mental or physical impairments are deemed to have 'needs' on that basis, and the condition of dementia itself is taken to define a category of people in need. The World Health Organisation distinguishes impairments from disabilities and handicaps.[1] An impairment occurs where people have a specific condition - some kind of 'anatomical, physiological or psychological abnormality or loss.'[2] A disability is the functional restriction which results from such a condition - the inability to perform certain tasks. A person whose disability causes disadvantage in a particular role or set of social roles is referred to as handicapped. The idea of 'dependency' is often used in relation to handicap; where disabled people are referred to as 'dependent' it usually indicates, not simply that they have certain functional problems, but that they have a dependent status. Needs can arise in relation to any of these categories, but they are needs of different kinds. Disability can be responded to by addressing the impairment, or by addressing the functional problems created by it - which implies either that a service is provided to help a person overcome functional limitations (e.g. reality orientation or occupational therapy) or that services themselves seek to overcome those limitations (e.g. the provision of meals and home helps). Handicap can in turn be responded to by addressing the impairment or the disability, or by seeking to change social relationships. This can mean the development or maintenance of relationships (in theory, one of the purposes of lunch clubs and day care); reducing social disadvantage (which can be achieved by providing services, and by offering special facilities like holidays); or compensating for that disadvantage by the development of alternative patterns of social life (e.g. through day care or residential care).

The needs of people with dementia

The kinds of problems experienced by people with dementia are complex. Dementia is defined (by Roth) as:

> a global deterioration of the individual's intellectual, emotional and conative faculties in a state of unimpaired consciousness.[3]

In order to establish the impact of dementia on a person's needs, it is important to distinguish the impairment from the functional problems it causes. The loss of intellectual faculties involves an inability to retain new information, and in consequence an inability to absorb it. This does not necessarily affect an individual's capacity for self or household care, but it may affect aspects of household management, including for example the ability to handle money, shop or plan meals. The loss of conative faculties - those concerned with self-direction and will - may affect both self and household care, as people become less able to maintain a routine, to distinguish day and night, or to understand events around them. It is difficult to say how far the deterioration of emotional faculties is part of the illness, and how far it is a response to the sense that 'something' is wrong. The effects may include strong expressions of emotion, including misplaced anger or sorrow, changes in behaviour, and consequent disruption of personal relationships, reinforced by the changes in capacity and behaviour which dementia implies.

At the same time, the problems which result from dementia are only a part of the kinds of problem which people with dementia may experience. Mental impairments are frequently experienced at the same time as other problems - including chronic physical illness, problems of mobility and continence - which are compounded by the kinds of problems which result from mental disorder. In addition, the consequences of dementia include not only changes in mental state, but also changes in social relationships. Often, these changes are exacerbated by other common changes experienced by elderly people, including the disruptions to communication caused by sensory impairments, the limited ability to participate in social activities which results from physical impairments or financial constraints, and the disruption of social relationships which are consequent on retirement and bereavement.

There is very little literature available on what it is like to experience dementia - not least because people with dementia are hardly ever asked. There are some creditable recent exceptions, most notably Kitwood and Bredin.[4] If people with dementia are able to answer, the assumption is likely to be made that they are not that demented; if they are not, it is only what one expects from people with dementia. There is a dangerous assumption concealed in this: that people with dementia have become a kind of human vegetable, incapable of reaction, feeling or normal emotion (a view reinforced because the disturbance of such responses is part of the diagnosis of the condition). But there are important reasons to question this view. Dementia is a progressive disease, and most people suffering from it retain social functioning to some degree. Kitwood and Bredin make a strong case that people with severe dementia are responsive to their social environment; even responses which are socially inappropriate (trying to clean up after incontinence with an item of clothing) still show a degree of social awareness, while in other cases there may be 'rementia' or a regaining of abilities through social interaction.

By contrast, the perspectives of carers are very well documented. Carers are often kin, often female and not uncommonly themselves elderly. The ability of carers to cope depends on many factors. Gilleard argues that it depends on the kinds of problems which are experienced, and not on the carers' perceptions of strain;[5] Zarit et al., by contrast, find that the perceived burden of carers, and not the degree of infirmity, is the main factor determining whether carers place people with dementia in nursing care.[6] The commitment of carers may be challenged by particular events or states: for example, sleep disturbance and faecal incontinence are particularly important in affecting the ability of carers to continue.[7] Jones also notes the importance of whether the burden of care falls on a single carer, rather than a number of people.[8]

It is difficult to say with confidence that the kinds of problems which are experienced are specific to dementia. Argyle et al. found that the problems most often reported were an inability to dress unaided, restlessness, urinary incontinence; from the point of view of the carers themselves, embarrassment, anxiety, and a decreased social life.[9] Gilleard argues that there are significant differences in the problems experienced by carers of geriatric and psychogeriatric patients. Some of these are predictable - geriatric patients, for example, are less likely to be able to get out of bed unaided, to be unsteady on their feet, or to be able to walk around the house, because loss of mobility is one of the primary reasons why they have been classified as geriatric patients. Psychogeriatric patients, conversely, are more likely to have behavioural problems.[10]

The problems of people with dementia are multi-faceted, and have to be understood in such terms. Gilleard et al. found that 'families of elderly mentally infirm patients perceive the problems of care in a multidimensional framework, reflecting dependency, behaviour disturbance, physical infirmity or disability, and emotional demands'.[11] Levin et al. argue that the experience of people with dementia and their carers has to be understood in terms of a number of dimensions: practical, behavioural, interpersonal, and social.[12] The range of needs, reflecting this range of problems, is similarly wide.

Responses to need

An implicit element in this discussion has been that needs have to be understood, not only in terms of problems, but also in terms of responses. People are thought of as being in need not simply because they have a problem, but because they are lacking something which will remedy that problem.[13] This means that needs must be needs for something. There are circumstances in which people with a degree of impairment have no identifiable 'needs' as a consequence: for example, some people with mild dementia continue to function normally in their own home,[14] and there may be no perception, either by the person with dementia or by carers, that there is any specific problem.[15] Pollitt et al. found that:

> a significant number of elderly dementia sufferers were being maintained in the community primarily by the care of the equally elderly spouses and that their use of assistance - both formal and informal- was much more limited than is often supposed.[16]

Problems have to be interpreted, or operationalised, as requiring a particular kind of response. Needs are often understood as needs for services - a need for housing, for medical care, for domestic support. 'It is easy', a recent government paper comments, 'to slip out of thinking "what does this person need?" into "what have we got that he/she could have?"'[17] The point is well made, but it is difficult, in practice, to avoid such an approach. Properly speaking, the definition of a 'need' is determined by the relationship between functional problems and possible responses.

This makes it difficult to establish precisely what services people need. There is often not just one possible response, but a range of options. People who are socially isolated might have that isolation reduced in a number of ways: for example, by introducing a number of people into their home, like voluntary visitors or even 'companions'; by bringing them into contact outside their home, through lunch clubs or day centres; and by changing the home, which is commonly done through sheltered housing or residential care. People who need housework done might have it done through domestic assistance, but they might also have it done through substitute family care or residential care. Strictly speaking, there can be no such thing as a 'need' for a lunch club or a home help; rather, there are needs which services of this kind may be able to satisfy to a greater or lesser degree. The assessment of needs is only a part of a wider process of service planning and provision; needs have to be interpreted in the light of the resources which are available.

The argument that needs concern such a relationship also implies that the interpretation of needs which people experience depends greatly on the resources which are available to them. Jones reviews the kinds of problems which predict whether or not elderly people with dementia are likely to be able to manage in the community. Favourable factors include a mild degree of mental illness; the presence of a sizeable, helpful family; the financial resources to cushion the situation; and the presence of support from community services. Conversely, adverse factors included the presence of severe illness, or disruptive behaviour; physical complications; an excessive burden of care falling on only one relative; a shortage of money; and a lack of support from professionals.[18] Blumenthal explains the importance of financial resources:

> if one has enough money, one can buy what one needs (e.g. companion, cook, housekeeper.) ... Until the dementia becomes profound, money can compensate for a good deal of functional deficit. One does not have to be able to cook, dial a phone number, to clean one's house, to go shopping, if there is no need to do so.[19]

If the issue is not so much that people have a problem, as that they do not have the resources to make adequate functioning possible, there is a case for concentrating attention on resource allocation rather than problems. Some commentators have argued that the idea of 'need' is redundant; it is more appropriate to consider the issue of demand.[20] A person who has a problem, and whose problem might be appropriately responded to by a particular service, does not necessarily present a demand to that service - a point which is of particular importance for people with dementia who may not accept that there is any reason to do anything. Conversely, there may be those who do demand services effectively - the demand for residential care is a case in point - even though they do not experience the appropriate problems or their problems are not best met by the responses available.

Needs and priorities

Even if services are directed to respond to demand rather than to need, there must be some way in which priorities between different kinds of demand can be established. The identification of 'need' constitutes a claim to service; the differentiation of various 'needs' distinguishes between people who are demanding services according to the strength of their claim.[21]

As part of a well-known 'taxonomy' of need, Bradshaw distinguishes normative, comparative, felt and expressed needs. Normative needs are those defined by experts; comparative, by comparison with others not in need; felt needs, those felt by the people themselves; and expressed, by the people or others in their name.[22] This classification touches on a range of issues; for our purposes here, there are two which are particularly important. One is the question of who defines the need; in the case of dementia, the people who have it are often unable to express need and sometimes are unaware of the severity of the problems they present.[23] The second, related issue is that some needs may be recognised, but not expressed. This poses a dilemma for planners: to what extent should provision be made for latent demand? The position is complicated by the processes through which demand is expressed: the demand often comes through referral by professionals after a non-specific request for service, so that the availability of particular options creates a channel or pattern of response to problems. To that extent, supply creates its own demand; and 'latent' demand is liable to become actual once services become available. Under-utilisation of services is conceivable - in the area of child care, for example, under-utilisation of residential facilities has become endemic, and in principle the same could happen in services for the elderly - but it is generally possible to adjust the levels of provision incrementally in order to make appropriate allowances.

An assessment of need is not equivalent to an allocations scheme; assessing need only provides decision makers with the kind of information which makes such decisions possible. The establishment of priorities depends on other considerations than needs alone.

Planning services for people with dementia

The objectives of services

Services for people with dementia can be understood in terms of several different objectives. The first order of objectives concerns issues of general principle, like the right to welfare, the development of the individual, or 'community care'. Community care, probably the most influential doctrine, has been concerned to maintain people in their own homes for as long as possible. But the idea of 'community care' is richly ambiguous. One celebrated distinction distinguishes care 'in' the community - which interprets the community as a geographical unit - from care 'by' the community, which understands communities in terms of a network of social relationships.[24] Within this broad categorisation, further subdivisions are possible.[25] Care 'in' the community might include any non-institutional care; care in 'ordinary housing' (the French term for 'community care' is 'le maintien à domicile', which at least has the virtue of honesty); or normalisation. Care 'by' the community might be understood as care by community services; care through the development of social networks; or care by informal carers, particularly families. These formulations do not imply one simple, unequivocal or uncontestable approach.

If a general aim of services is to make it possible for people to continue in 'the community' for as long as possible, it is unclear whether provision of services appropriate to people's needs will achieve that end. Gilhooly writes:

> For some time it was assumed that care for dementing old people "broke down", and supporters then requested or demanded institutional care. Furthermore, it was assumed that, if some of the problems of giving care in the community could be alleviated by providing services, supporters would continue to give care. Research evidence to date, however, calls into question such assumptions.[26]

The evidence considered is not unequivocal; if people who receive more care are more likely to move to institutional care, it may be because their needs are more serious,[27] and not because the services significantly affect the ability of carers to cope, positively or negatively. Gilhooly comments that:

> formal services as currently provided do not prevent institutionalisation; nor do they do a lot to reduce burden or distress. This may be because not enough is provided in the way of services, or because the types of services provided are not appropriate.[28]

It seems difficult, in the current state of knowledge, to base any decisions on the likely advantages of particular policies in promoting maintenance at home. This should not, however, be taken to undermine the justification for providing services in people's homes; the provision of many services is defensible, much more simply, in terms of promoting welfare and improving the quality of life.

Second-order objectives concern the method of meeting these broad aims, which imply the setting of specific goals, such as improving functional capacities or the meeting of domiciliary needs. Specific goals may be operationalised (that is, translated into practicable terms) and met fairly directly. One view, reflecting the 'rational' approach to planning,[29] is that planners should seek, through the matching of need or demand to services, to maximise the achievement of goals at the minimum expense - 'cost-effectiveness'.[30] An alternative view, which reflects an 'incremental' approach, is that planners should be trying, within constraints, progressively to adjust the level of services provided to need.[31] This would be compatible with the kind of care management envisaged in the Griffiths report,[32] which sees the role of service planners primarily in terms of developing a range of services from which an individually tailored package of provision can be selected by a case manager. Etzioni advocates 'mixed scanning', a combination of such approaches, for the best results.[33]

There are, in addition, third-order objectives. These include efficiency - the reduction of unit cost, or the elimination of waste - and cost-containment.[34] They are 'third order' because they imply the imposition of constraints on pre-existing objectives, rather than constituting fundamental objectives in themselves.

Services for people with dementia

There are many different kinds of service available for people with dementia. Many of the services can be seen as alternatives, even if they are not directly equivalent. A person who cannot prepare a meal may, for example, receive meals on wheels or attend a lunch club; a person who requires supervision at night may enter residential care or have a night sitter; someone who needs supportive social contact may be offered substitute family care or day care. These services do not offer the same kind of care on the same terms, and where they exist in conjunction with each other it should be possible to establish criteria by which one person might be considered to need one service while another person should receive another. Where the services do not all exist, however, they may be used as substitutes for each other.

This makes it difficult to establish what the 'need' is for any particular service. Needs are not formed in a social vacuum; people look for the response which is most appropriate, which is available, and which is feasible. New options - like 'very sheltered' housing, care and repair, night sitting or elderly fostering - often become possible, although they are not very generally practised; other options, like nursing care, may be well established but are not necessarily the most appropriate option. The way that needs are operationalised depends on the context in which services operate: if people cannot be considered to 'need' three baths a week, even if many people would have taken at least that many before coming infirm, it is because there is no practical way to provide them with the support which is necessary. Concepts of need within agencies are formed in the light of practical constraints.[35]

Norman lists the community care services which are most directly concerned with people with dementia as:

- general practitioners
- social workers
- community-based nursing services
- home helps
- intensive home care services
- incontinence services
- night sitters

- voluntary sitting-in schemes
- boarding out schemes
- bought in services (obtained on an ad hoc basis)
- voluntary counselling services, and
- relatives' support groups.[36]

Other services, such as hospital care, day care and residential care clearly have a large role to play. Some of the services Norman mentions are very infrequently encountered - her book is in part a plea for the establishment of a wider range of services; but the list is as surprising for the services it omits as for those it includes. Among those omitted, Melzer et al. include:

- occupational therapists
- health visitors
- wardens of sheltered housing
- transport
- paramedical services - optics, dentistry, chiropody, audiometry family break schemes, and
- social security,[37]

while others still are not included on either list, like staying put schemes or substitute family care.

The main services available to people with dementia are classified by Melzer et al. in eight groups:

- screening and early recognition
- assessment and treatment (medical and social)
- dementia therapies
- information and counselling
- community support substitution service (e.g. meals, transport)
- respite care
- financial help, and
- long term residential care.

These categories overlap to some degree, both because the organisation of some services links assessment with specific responses, and because the same services can offer alternative treatments.[38]

The current pattern of provision for elderly people with dementia seems, in general, to be one in which the level of all services received remains fairly constant, irrespective of the severity of the dementia.[39] This finding is at first sight puzzling; the basic explanation is that people with or without dementia have a range of needs, including problems with mobility, self care and household care, which are more important in determining the overall level of service given. If an assessment is made primarily on the basis of physical or functional dependency, the relationship between services and needs is much stronger.[40] O'Connor et al. suggest that the kinds of services allocated - commonly home helps and meals on wheels - have limited applicability to the situation of old people living with relatives, but that other services which might be more appropriate, like home nursing or day hospital, have a limited coverage. There are many alternative ways of providing for similar problems: under 'dementia therapies', for example, Melzer et al. list reality orientation, cognitive stimulation, validation therapy and drug therapies.

Decisions which are made about the provision of particular services have to take into account the status quo, available resources, the feasibility of introducing different kinds of option, and the perceived desirability of different options. A working party on sheltered housing, for example, has argued that sheltered housing is not a suitable option for people with dementia: they suggest that it is potentially disruptive to collective living arrangements, and consequently 'positively disadvantageous for the sick person'.[41] There are grounds to question such a view. Sheltered housing can be used positively for people with milder dementias, in order to provide supervision or social contact; and if the problem is that dementia is disruptive to communal living, the objection to placing people in residential or nursing care must be much stronger. The evidence on the value of alarm systems for people with dementia is inconclusive.[42] But even if the argument that sheltered housing was unsuitable was accepted, it would not follow that the service should not be included within service planning. People with dementia will use sheltered housing, if only because people may develop dementia while they are there. It will meet at least some of their needs, and so it will affect the level of demand for other kinds of service. It will have to be used as a substitute when other services are not available. The test of a measure of the needs of a population is not that it leads to the right kind of prescription for provision, but that it helps to identify the kinds of consideration on which the planning of services can be based.

Challis points to a number of problems associated with planning for the existing range of services: the growing numbers of elderly people requiring help exceed the resources of services to deal with them, needs and services often do not match, services are fragmented, and they are often unco-ordinated at the level of the individual.[43] The assessment of needs can assist with planning services in the first place by identifying problems for which responses are required, and secondly by helping to define the role that services are expected to take in relation to those needs. However, it cannot of itself improve co-ordination, or prevent fragmentation of services; and although it may improve the match between needs and services, there is no guarantee that the use of services will be more appropriate.

The role of planners

Planning is not a simple, uncontested area of work, and the purpose of needs assessment for use by planners could be understood in several different ways. Needs assessment can be seen, simply, as the identification of needs as a basis for the allocation of resources. But it would be consistent with alternative views of the planning process to present the role of needs assessment in other terms. A basic distinction needs to be made between the planner as provider and that of enabler. Planning in the health service has primarily been directed to provision; by contrast, the planning of community care, which is now being led by Social Services/ Social Work Departments, depends formally on a view of state provision as ancillary to existing support networks. Because the roles of planners overlap and vary, it seems appropriate to try and ensure that the methods used are adaptable to each of these purposes. This implies consideration of both individual cases, and an overview of problems; and the identification both of the full range of possible responses, and the kinds of responses which can be made available in particular cases.

Service priorities

The main purpose of assessing needs in planning is to provide information as a basis for deciding what should be provided, and how much of it should be provided. This is not quite the same as a statement about which needs can be met, and which cannot. Meeting needs requires an allocation of resources; all needs are not equal. In conditions where resources are scarce, the needs which are met are (or at least should be) those to which the greatest priority has been given. But even where resources are relatively plentiful - as, for example, when services are intended to expand - the relative nature of different needs implies that as some classes of needs are met others, of a lesser order, come to the fore. Needs are not, then, simply present or absent; they are also of greater or lesser priority.

The identification of needs does not in itself determine specific priorities. What it should provide is basic information on which allocations can subsequently be based. Allocations concern decisions about inputs rather than about outputs. Planners meet needs only indirectly; the kind of decision that will generally be made is to provide aids and adaptations and home helps, not to provide generic services for people with mild dementia without social support or for people with moderate dementia and some restriction of physical abilities. But the kind of information provided by a needs assessment is usually of the latter kind, rather than the former. It is important, then, to provide some kind of method through which information about needs can be translated into information about the demand for services. One has then to match the kinds of problem which are identified with the kinds of services which are available. This does not mean that every person's need for particular services has to be assessed, but the kinds of problems which are identified have to include those which will constitute the basis of the allocation of the services. This implies, in turn, that the process of assessing need has to be conceived in terms which can subsequently be applied to the criteria applied for the allocation of services.

3 The assessment of needs

Measuring needs

Needs are often nebulous: aims like an 'independent life in the community' or 'personal development' are too vague to be operationalised directly. An instrument intended to measure needs of a population has to begin with second-order objectives, like physical capacity, personal care or household management. Even this kind of aim may be difficult to translate into measurable terms; at best, instruments offer an indication of the issues, rather than a definitive statement.

Criteria for measurement

The standard tests of such an instrument concern validity, reliability and ease of application. There are at least two more factors which should also be considered: adaptability and robustness.

Validity An instrument is valid to the extent that it measures the problem or problems that it is supposed to measure. This is difficult to guarantee, because the process of operationalisation itself demands that some compromises are made: if it is not possible either to consider higher-order objectives in their own right, or directly to link functional problems to possible responses, the instrument can only offer an insight into the total process, rather than an authoritative answer to planners' questions.

Reliability Instruments are reliable if they yield consistent results in similar circumstances when applied by different people. The advantage of consistency is that, even if the instrument is not an ideal reflection of the problem being studied, one can at least get some feeling for the relative seriousness of a problem, or of the effect of changes over time. An instrument is likely to be used in a variety of settings, by people with a range of different skills. It should not, ideally, yield very different results when administered by a social work assistant, a nurse, a residential care worker; it should not, then, be dependent on the professional skills or background of staff.

Ease of application and use Validity and reliability can both be improved to some degree by using a battery of different techniques of analysis. There are, however, important practical limitations. Kane and Kane suggest three main criteria: minimising the time and cost of administration; minimising the cost of analysis; and minimising the equipment required.[1] It should be possible to administer an instrument within a reasonable period of time (because longer interviews create fatigue in the parties and lead to unreliability, and long instruments encourage those administering them to cut corners). Conversely, at the planning end, an instrument which can only be used by people with a medical qualification and a Master's degree in Operational Research will have limited applicability.

Adaptability Planning is not a simple, unitary activity; and local planning seeks to define options and approaches over a range of services, geographical areas and patterns of client need. An instrument which is designed for local planning has to be adaptable to the full range of circumstances in which it is likely to be applied. Because these circumstances change, the instrument has also to be adaptable over time.

Robustness A related issue is that of 'robustness' (the term is drawn from the literature on operational research): the selection of options in conditions of uncertainty which do least to limit potential outcomes. In practice, an instrument of this kind is likely to be used in a wide variety of contexts. Irrespective of the qualifications which might be made about its use, if it offers a convenient means of assessment it will be used for want of anything better in circumstances where a degree of caution might be called for. It seems clear that any instrument which can be applied to individual cases is liable to be used for individual assessments. But an instrument which is to be used for planning purposes is not the same as one which might serve for individual assessment. An instrument of that type would require assessment of each individual's circumstances; categorisation of symptoms in terms which allow the figures to be used in different ways; elimination of undesired alternatives; and specification of the context in which diagnosis is taking place. Instruments used for planning, by contrast, permit approximation - because errors in aggregate should cancel each other out; the classification of problems should be grouped according to response; and the instruments should be capable of producing results at different levels of aggregation. Ideally, instruments which are used for different purposes should be different; but as a compromise it is probably better to have an instrument which is capable of being adapted to different purposes than it is to depend on tools which are wholly task-specific but which can only be used effectively in narrowly defined circumstances.

Other criteria, like plausibility and sensitivity to circumstances, might also reasonably be applied.

The use of indicators

The kinds of assessment with which an instrument for planning must deal are not 'facts'. The assessment of needs requires a series of judgments to be made: about the people who should be assessed, about the kinds of factors which need to be taken into account, and the situation of the people who are undergoing assessment. The process is not 'subjective', in the sense of relying solely on individual assessors, but nor is it 'objective' in the sense of being clear, value-free, unambiguous, or a simple exercise in counting. What an instrument can reasonably provide is a much more modest statement, in the form of 'indicators'.[2] An indicator is a signpost rather than an unequivocal statement of fact; much of the value of producing indicators is that, even if some compromises have been necessary on the way, the comparison of indicators over time gives at least some clue as to whether problems continue or change, or (in the case of service provision) if they have been alleviated or aggravated. It is important, for this reason, to provide an instrument which reproduces results fairly reliably, but at the same time the instrument must be able to cope with uncertainty and ambiguity, without relying on too many limiting assumptions which may prove to be untenable in practice.

The kinds of judgments which have to be made in order to assess need are necessarily qualitative: they rely on an appraisal of a situation rather than the identification of facts which are present or not. Necessarily, for the purposes of planning it is important to systematise and regularise the kinds of judgement which are made. However, it is important not to lose sight of the kinds of data with which one is working; and the effect of seeking to treat such judgments as if they were quantifiable 'facts' may be to assume a regularity and homogeneity in the material which is not justifiable in practice. The assumption that material can be quantified requires that factors can be homogenised - so that one factor, like behaviour, can meaningfully be related to another, like self-care; and that factors can be aggregated, so that two factors are greater than one. Neither assumption is necessarily justified, and there is a risk that the quantification of an erratic variable can inject a serious or persistent bias into results and render them meaningless.

The needs of a population

The process of planning for a population is not the same as planning to meet the needs of specific individuals. In planning for a population, people are being dealt with in aggregate. The needs and circumstances of individuals may change, but the needs of populations generally change much more slowly (because fluctuations cancel each other out). The position of the 'average' person in a population of elderly people is very unlike that of any real individual. The 'average' person in an elderly population moves infrequently, and does not move out of an area; she does not suffer major upheavals or catastrophes; and she never dies. This kind of assumption, common in economic reasoning, is effectively built into the process of planning for a population. The individuals whose needs are identified at one point of time are not necessarily those for whom resources are provided at another; but information about the status quo is usually the best information available about the potential pattern of needs in the future.

The population with dementia is less stable than the population of elderly people overall. The point at which 'dementia' might be said to have begun is difficult to define with any certainty; as a progressive disorder, people with dementia pass through different levels of need, though the likely impact of the progress of dementia on social functioning has never been very clearly defined; and there is a higher rate of mortality than in the rest of the elderly population. The term 'population' is itself liable to be misleading, because there is no constant group of people. What there is is a flow of people, which creates an identifiable pool whose needs have to be responded to at any one point in time.

Incidence Although there has been a substantial amount of research into the epidemiology of dementia, many points remain unclear. Estimates of prevalence depend greatly on the definition of the disease, with the greatest uncertainty concerning those who experience only mild dementia.[3] Incidence, because of the slow onset of the disease, is even more difficult to gauge, though Henderson cites a number of studies.[4] Copeland et al. estimate annual rates of 9.2 per 1000 over the age of 65, ranging from 3.8 aged 65-74 to 28.7 over the age of 85.[5] An annual figure of 15.4 per 1000 over 65 was found in a study in Mannheim in Germany.[6] The Gospel Oak Study suggests a higher figure again, of 26 per 1000 over the age of 65, ranging from 8 per 1000 aged 65-69 to 22 per 1000 aged 70-79 and 39 per 1000 for those over 80.[7]

Mortality. The available information on mortality also shows wide variation between studies. Copeland et al. estimate 19% per annum.[8] Jorm et al. found 82% mortality over 5 years,[9] suggesting an annual mortality rate of approximately 29%. Our returns following the census of people with dementia in Angus[10] suggest a mortality rate equivalent to 23% p.a.; this may be an underestimate, because we were unable to track deaths among those newly admitted to long-stay hospital from the community.

The flow of people with dementia

Information about the survival and movement of people with dementia is markedly lacking, but it is possible from the figures on incidence and prevalence to construct an initial model of the flow of the population of dementia sufferers through dementia. Putting figures for incidence together with prevalence gives some initial indication of patterns for the population with dementia. On EURODEM figures, 69 people in 1000 aged 65 or over in Scotland suffer from dementia; an incidence of between 15 and 20 per 1000 suggests an influx of between 22% and 29%.

The likely distribution of people with dementia between community and institutions can be estimated at roughly 60:40. Dementia is a progressive disease, and people are likely to go from mild dementia through to severe dementia unless death intervenes. This progression may imply a move from community to institutional care, and although there are other kinds of move (community-community, institution-institution and institution-community) this is the most likely pattern of movement.

The position of people with dementia changes fairly rapidly. Goda followed up psychogeriatric referrals (which would include some conditions other than dementia) and found at an interval of 32 weeks that 51% were still at home, 25% were in institutions, 12% were dead, and 13% were unknown.[11] Knopman et al. found, in a small sample with 'advanced dementia', that in a two year period 23% died and 29% moved to nursing homes.[12] In the follow-up to the Angus census, which is reported more fully later in this book, 77 people out of 278 had moved to institutions in a 236 day period, suggesting an annual movement of over 40%. In the census in Dundee, also reported later, 75 people out of 398 transferrred to institutional care in a period of 123 days, which implies an annual rate of over 50%. Those going into hospital cannot confidently be identified as movers, because some would subsequently return home, some would go into other forms of care and some would die; there may also have been some mortality shortly after moving to institutional care, which we were not in a position to identify. The indications are, however, that well over a third of the people in the community with recognised dementia may move to institutions in the course of a year. Our sample was probably biased towards those in the community whose dementia was more severe, and this estimate needs to be treated with caution, but this does suggest a rapid turnover.

It is difficult to be precise about such outcomes, which would necessitate a longitudinal study. It is possible, however, to approach the problem in theoretical terms, modelling the flow under certain assumptions, and then seeking to examine the consequences of those assumptions.

On the basis of the literature and our work in Tayside, it is not implausible to assume

- that 60% of the people with dementia are in community care, and 40% in residential care;
- that the incidence of dementia relative to the existing population is 24% per annum;
- that incidence primarily occurs in the community;
- that annually, 15% of people with dementia in the community die;
- that 25% of those in the community transfer each year to institutions;
- and that 37.5% of those in institutions die.

Table 3.1
The flow of people with dementia

	Year 0	Year 1	Year 2	Year 3	Year 4
Community care					
Initial pool	60	36	22	16	11
Year 1 incidence		24	14	8	5
Year 2 incidence			22	14	8
Year 3 incidence				22	14
Year 4 incidence					22
Total	60	60	60	60	60
Residential/institutional care					
Initial pool	40	25	16	10	6
Year 1 intake		15	9	6	4
Year 2 intake			15	9	6
Year 3 intake				15	9
Year 4 intake					15
Total	40	40	40	40	40

This implies overall mortality of 24%, and a stable prevalence. Table 3.1 describes the flow in a pool of 100 people. Only 61% of people are likely to be in the same position after one year, and 38% after two. This does not include those whose position in the community has deteriorated.

The effect of the assumptions is as follows:

- The effect of higher mortality would be to increase the rate of change: mortality of 29%, depending on its distribution between community and residential care, would bring the figures for those remaining in the same position down to 56% after one year and 31% after 2. Conversely, lower mortality of 19% would lower the rate of change, with 66% remaining after year 1 and 45% after year 2.
- Since 40% of the people in community care have been assumed to change circumstances each year, by comparison with 37.5% in residential care, a higher proportion of people in community care would have the effect of marginally increasing the rate of change. If the balance of mortality alters between community and residential care, or the rate of transfer to residential care alters - either of which could be brought about through altering the availability of residential care - the relative figures for residential and community care could alter considerably. The balance between residential and community care is in consequence not a robust assumption.
- A decrease in the rate of transfer to residential care would reduce the rate of change, but in so far as this represented different treatment for people with needs that would otherwise have been met in residential care, this would partially be offset by increased mortality in the community.

There are, of course, many weaknesses in the assumptions.

- The size of the pool is not constant; the assumptions made here are intended to produce a balanced flow, with mortality equal to incidence. The age structure of a locality is liable to vary. Incidence has shown no change in recent years,[13] though it has been suggested that it may fall.[14] Greater incidence combined with lesser mortality generally would reduce the speed of the flow; greater mortality and lesser incidence would increase it.
- Fluctuations in the characteristics of the population do not necessarily cancel each other out; the smaller the population under consideration, the less convincing the assumption of a smooth flow is likely to be.
- Dementia is not neatly progressive.
- Institutional care is not necessarily offered at a later stage in the progress of dementia than community care.

Despite these limitations, the model does point to some important issues from the point of view of planners.

- There is no constant 'population with dementia' for whom plans are being made.
- Changes in the circumstances of people with dementia tend to take place over a short period of time. On a range of assumptions, most people reviewed at any one point of time will be in a different position after two years. That means that projects for service response which take this long from conception to implementation - which probably includes most new projects - are necessarily addressed principally not to the problems of people who have dementia now, but to problems which are likely to arise in the future.
- For planning purposes, there is only a limited advantage in trying to develop more accurate returns in relation to problems which cannot be responded to directly, because circumstances change so rapidly. In important respects refinement and greater accuracy in assessing needs may be misleading to planners; plans have to be generalised across a population, and precise assessments in relation to a particular cohort do not necessarily reflect the needs of the population in the future.

Some implications for services should also be noted.

- People who have dementia over a long period of time in stable circumstances are untypical - only one-sixth of the initial pool in the model can be expected to be in the same circumstances after four years. To respond to problems effectively, services need to be geared to people who may have problems for relatively short periods, and to be sufficiently flexible to respond to changes in circumstances.
- Delays in implementation can be expected to have a devastating effect on the potential benefit for any current cohort.
- There is little practical prospect of achieving continuity through the operation of any service in isolation; there may be a case for a nominated key contact of the kind used elsewhere in community services.

4 The development of the profile

The matrix approach

Because we were seeking to develop an instrument which could be worked with at different levels, the data it produced had to be capable of being aggregated or disaggregated flexibly. This meant that the kind of instrument which we intended to develop had to be based on small units of assessment - and so, for practical purposes, on individual assessments. It did not have to be accurate in every detail, because it was providing a set of indicators rather than the kind of assessment which is necessary for the management of individual cases; but it did have to be sufficiently detailed and flexible to permit use in a variety of ways for planning purposes.

The problems of quantitative assessments

Several instruments of this kind have been based principally on quantitative data. Wilkin argues:

> The needs of those responsible for the formulation of policy and its implementation through the provision of health and welfare services demand simple measurement instruments which yield results amenable to aggregation and classification. But these simple instruments may distort an extremely complex reality.[1]

The use of quantitative statistical techniques offers a powerful tool for the analysis of data, but there are serious reservations about the application of such techniques to the kinds of problems under review. In principle, the use of multivariate analysis makes it possible to differentiate between factors according to their influence in determining priority for services. Where factors commonly occur together, the use of appropriate statistical methods (like a stepwise multiple regression analysis) allows the user to select from a range of contributing factors those which have most effect in shaping the pattern of use. There are four main problems with such an approach. In the first place, the results which are produced are derived from empirical experience rather than from principle, and there is a danger that the resulting model will be insensitive to changing circumstances or may enshrine present practice. Secondly, the process implies the establishment of statistical norms, and exceptional cases ('outliers') are excluded from the analysis; the results are not likely to be sensitive to unusual circumstances. Third, the assumptions which have to be made about the mathematical relationship of factors are often questionable, particularly in view of the very uncertain nature of much of the data; and multivariate analysis is particularly vulnerable to distortion by one highly unreliable element in the analysis. Lastly, the results of such an analysis are often implausible, because in their very nature they imply the exclusion of relevant factors in the interests of simplifying and summarising circumstances.

The use of 'points schemes', like the Behavioural Rating Scale of the CAPE[2] or the Crichton Royal Behavioural Rating scale,[3] offers a compromise between the strict quantitative measurement demanded as a basis for multivariate analysis and freer-ranging qualitative data. Points schemes allow the construction of indicators of need which are, whatever their limitations, at least able to distinguish between varying circumstances and fairly consistent in their treatment of values. The problems which exist in such scales can be summarised as follows. First, there is the problem of inclusion - that they may include items which are inappropriate to the purpose - and exclusion, that they may exclude other factors which are relevant. The way in which these problems can most effectively be overcome is by seeking to provide a reasonably comprehensive measure from which items can be dropped as necessary, or to which supplementary scales can be added, without distorting the balance of the elements which have been maintained. (This is virtually impossible in any scheme derived from a regression equation.) Second, there is the problem of weighting, so that factors play a role appropriate to their relative importance. This is problematic in a number of scales; in the Crichton Royal scale, for example, non-cooperation with staff is given as much weight as mobility incapacity. Third, there is the issue of quantification in itself. The attachment of numbers to factors implies that they can be added together or subtracted from each other - which is not necessarily the case in service provision. Small factors may continue to require individuated responses; large factors may not require a larger response; and different constellations of problem may require, not greater responses, but different categories of response. Lastly, the instrument has to be adapted to the purposes for which it is intended - which means, in this case, that it provides information about the needs for a variety of service delivered by different agencies.

These kinds of problems have led us to seek to develop an instrument which avoids precise quantification; which establishes a profile or matrix of needs, to be aggregated or disaggregated as necessary, rather than constructing a single aggregate score; and which, while trying to be reasonably comprehensive, will be adaptable to a range of needs.

Developing a matrix

An instrument which meets these requirements can be expected to have multiple dimensions, rather than a uniform scale. Dementia is strongly associated with a range of problems, including locomotor difficulties, self-care and disturbed behaviour.[4] The CAPE scale was developed from four distinct areas of functional disability: physical disability, apathy, communication difficulties and social disturbance.[5] The effect of aggregating results, however, is often to lose sight of the component problems. The construction of a matrix makes it possible to discriminate finely between different categories of cases while maintaining the appearance of simplicity. An example of this approach is Thompson's work on assessing the needs of elderly people for residential care.[6] Thompson distinguishes three main categories of need: physical (P), mental (M) and social (S). In each category, old people are judged against a simple scale (e.g. S1, S2, S3); Thompson identifies four grades of physical need, seven relating to social factors and seven relating to mental state. The possible combinations of need are then classified according to priority (for example, P1/M3/S2 ranks above P3/M3/S4). Although the principle behind the categorisation is fairly basic, the use of three categories with a number of grades still offer 196 possible combinations (that is, 4 x 7 x 7). The situations a dementia planning instrument has to deal with are very much more diverse than those determining admission to residential care, but it is simple enough to increase the sensitivity of this kind of approach, either by increasing the number of dimensions or by refining the system of ranking. Using six dimensions with five grades, for example, creates 15,625 possible combinations - which, in principle, should be more than enough if the right kind of factors are selected.

The basic dimensions of the matrix have to identify a range of issues and problems which together will form a profile of a person's needs, but which can be aggregated or disaggregated in different ways in order to provide information relevant to service provision and planning. What the matrix approach offers is a powerful basis on which to assess needs while respecting the kinds of consideration which have been outlined so far. The use of qualitative rather than quantitative data allows for a sensitive and adaptable approach without having to rely on the kinds of heroic assumption which bedevil the construction of indices. The matrix permits the use of related factors in order to provide information for different purposes.

Identifying functional problems gives only one part of the information necessary to identify needs. This has to be set against existing support, both informal and formal, to identify gaps and mismatches. A key element in the approach to meeting needs is the idea that different functional problems, and patterns of problems, can be met through a range of alternative services. By preserving the data on which such judgments are made, and allowing the information to be reconstructed in a range of different ways, it is possible to examine the implications of different patterns of service on the range of functional problems. Within the profiles, it should be possible to identify those kinds of cases in which the allocation of particular kinds of service - like home helps or district nursing - are considered important, and with what degree of priority they are to be considered. The approach does not guarantee a definitive answer, but it establishes a regularised set of information which can be drawn upon in different ways for different purposes.

Building the matrix

The component dimensions of the matrix focus on the identification of functional problems. The use of the matrix approach creates, for each person examined, a profile - that is, a composite picture of need - while at the same time permitting consideration of specific dimensions discretely.

Constructing a matrix depends on two basic elements. The first calls for the identification of the dimensions of the matrix - the categories of need which are being considered. Given the arguments which have been made about need, this has to refer primarily to functional problems, which can be gauged in relation to the available responses. The second task is to develop some means of ranking information within each dimension. This calls again for a functional classification, which can be applied to the demand for services, rather than a simple test of severity.

The starting point for considering the dimensions of need was the categorisation of dependency developed by Bond and Carstairs.[7] This has five 'components of dependency':

- mobility
- self-care
- house care
- incontinence, and
- mental state.

The first three are based on functional criteria - the ability of the individual to perform certain basic tasks. They were incorporated into the profile as mobility, personal care and domestic tasks. The other two were modified: incontinence was dealt with as an aspect of personal care, and mental state, because it is not directly indicative of needs, was replaced by a dimension relating to behaviour requiring intervention. Further dimensions were added referring to material needs and the needs of carers.

Within categories, the measure that has to be used concerns the implications of the need, rather than its severity; the severity of a functional problem is not necessarily a guide to the kind of response which is required. Finklestein, criticising the OPCS studies of disability, gives an illustration of this: it is not necessarily true that being in a wheelchair implies a more severe functional restriction of mobility than being able to walk only 50 yards, because the wheelchair makes certain kinds of mobility possible.[8] What is required is not an index of severity, but rather some measure of the need for a response - assistance, intervention or active watchfulness.

The approach taken by Isaacs and Neville[9] was to identify levels of functional need in terms of the time during which an individual could cope without aid or attention. This provides the clearest indication of the level of commitment required by services or informal carers to respond to the core areas of need defined by the main dimensions of the profile: mobility, personal care, domestic tasks, behaviour.

The 'intervals' defined by Isaacs and Neville were:

Critical interval	Attention needed at short and unpredictable intervals.
Short interval	Attention needed more than once a day at times which can be arranged (eg meal times).
Long interval	Attention needed not more than once a day.
Independent	No need.

Bond and Carstairs[10] extended Isaacs and Neville's scheme. They defined seven levels of dependency, two of which were repetitions of other levels with the additional factor of mental disorder. Short interval need was divided into two categories: day only, and night and day. The Tayside Profile returns to Isaacs and Neville's simpler original, but with separate sub-dimensions covering night attention for personal care and behaviour.

Bond and Carstairs developed a set of specific questions relating to task performance which were used to define the interval level of need. We attempted initially to use these tasks as examples, but respondents tended to focus too much on the specific named tasks without considering the overall level of need for assistance. This led to the present format, where respondents are required to assess directly the interval into which a subject should be placed.

This 'interval' categorisation of levels of need applies to mobility, personal care, domestic tasks and behaviour; it is also used to classify the involvement of carers, which can be seen both as a response to need and as a need in itself. Other needs which were included in the profile - material needs, solitude and the subjective problems of caring - did not fit these categories. Their definitions are outlined in the discussion of factors which follows.

The dimensions of the profile

We have called the instrument which was developed the Tayside Profile for Dementia Planning. The profile is based on seven main dimensions:

- Mobility
- Personal care
- Domestic tasks
- Behaviour
- Solitude
- Material needs, and
- The needs of carers.

This section describes each of these dimensions in more detail.

Mobility This dimension is about the physical ability to move around, and is identified in terms of the profile's standard categories of need. The emphasis on intervention means that the test is strictly functional; people need some kind of intervention or support when they cannot manage by themselves, not simply because they have problems with mobility.

The issue of mobility needs, for this purpose, to be distinguished from orientation. People who do not walk, or who are unable to orient themselves, have problems with mobility, but the kinds of problems they have and the kinds of intervention they require are generally related to the pattern of behaviour rather than their functional capacity. Because different kinds of intervention are required in those circumstances, this is classified in the profile as a behavioural issue rather than a problem of mobility.

Personal care This dimension concerns the ability to undertake the basic functions of bodily maintenance, including continence. It is identified in terms of the profile's standard categories of need. A separate category records the need for assistance with personal care at night. The need for assistance or prompting to take medicine appropriately is also included in the personal care dimension.

Incontinence was incorporated within the dimension of personal care, because the response to incontinence is in many cases equivalent to issues relating to personal care, and support is often given on the same terms. There is no question that incontinence is an important issue in its own right,[11] but our focus was on functional need rather than specific problematic conditions, and it was decided to incorporate it rather than to treat it as a separate dimension. Many night needs and critical interval needs relate to continence problems. Continence may be achieved, particularly in residential and hospital settings, by frequent prompting or toileting. Such actions count as assistance and are coded to the appropriate level of need. The same applies to the changing of continence devices such as pads. Night care includes assistance to and from the toilet, even if no intimate assistance is required.

In some cases the need for help with personal care in informal settings, as well as for domestic tasks, might come about because a carer thinks that the person with dementia cannot manage adequately, and not because the sufferer cannot actually manage.[12] For example, the person with dementia might be able to dress without assistance, but not to a standard acceptable to the carer.

Domestic Tasks This dimension includes the basic tasks of household maintenance and preparation of food and drink. It was identified in terms of the profile's standard categories of need. However, there is no critical interval category since there is no need for assistance with domestic tasks at that level of intensity.

There was some debate as to whether the ability to perform domestic tasks was an appropriate question to ask in residential, nursing and hospital care; residents usually have little scope to demonstrate their ability at domestic tasks. It is impossible to identify whether there is any scope to meet needs in alternative ways without having information about the capacities of the person with dementia.

Behaviour This dimension includes all manifestations of behavioural abnormality that require the attention or assistance of a carer - a set of problems which has been described as central to what sets dementia apart from other conditions.[13] Some scales conflate behaviours and issues relating to the relationships of people with dementia and their carers: 'co-operativeness', for example, which occurs in the CAPE scale, depends on the behaviour of the carer as well as the person with dementia. It is difficult to avoid this altogether, because the principal informants are certain to describe the way the person they are caring for responds to them.

There are many studies of behaviour problems in dementia. The kinds of problem described include behaviours which require the carer's attention and vigilance, such as wandering, nocturnal activity, dangerous activity; emotionally trying behaviours, such as aggression, abuse, accusations, excessive dependency or attention-demanding; and inappropriate micturition and faecal disposal.[14]

We investigated the possibility of trying to align Greene's Behaviour and Mood Disturbance Scale,[15] which is based on such factors, with the interval level of measurement. This scale defines behaviour as withdrawn or apathetic, active mood disturbance and disturbed behaviour. It seemed at first that we could, in rough terms, regard withdrawn or apathetic behaviour as equivalent to long-interval need, more active (or troublesome) mood disturbance as short-interval need and disturbed behaviour as critical-interval need. In practice it proved to be not so simple. Apathy could involve self-neglect - e.g. inadequate meals - which would imply short-interval need. Greene's scale focused attention on particular behaviours rather than on the level of intervention needed. After experimenting with this, we found it better to define behaviour needs simply in terms of the standard time-based levels of intervention.

The level of need is, then, identified in terms of the profile's standard categories of need. This has two distinct advantages over other evaluations. The first is that the test depends less on any judgment of the quality of the behaviour than on the question of whether behaviour requires intervention. (This might include apathy and withdrawal.) The second is that it identifies the need which arises in terms of the time required of carers, which is the basis on which any service response has to be gauged.

Solitude Social interaction is an important aspect of human life. Dementia does not diminish its importance, even if it distorts and disrupts the ability of the person with dementia to participate in social interaction, or show evidence of benefit. This is an important consideration for services which provide such contact; the decision to send someone to a lunch club, or to recommend group living, is often influenced by an assessment of the patterns of social contact. As well as a basic question on whether the person with dementia lives alone or not, the profile includes a rating of solitude, based on the time the person with dementia spends at home alone during a typical day. It may of course be true that people are not alone, but still do not interact with others; the best we can aim to do is to look for situations in which interaction is possible.

The inspiration for this was Isaacs and Neville's[16] solitude rating, but there is an important conceptual difference. Isaacs and Neville used solitude as an indicator of support; we were concerned with the maintenance of social contact. It follows that isolation during the night does not have the significance it has in Isaacs and Neville's rating.

Material Needs Material needs and material resources are two sides of the same coin. The material resources which are of the greatest practical importance are money (income and capital), housing and material possessions.

Although in principle it should be easy to identify financial resources and needs, there are in practice a number of technical and practical problems, not least the sensitivity which surrounds financial matters, which suggest this area should be approached indirectly. Likewise, it is not practicable to work through in detail all possible needs relating to housing and material possessions. This calls for the use of indicators as a practical alternative to the precise measurement of needs and resources.

No indicator of material needs and resources is wholly satisfactory. It would be helpful to know the actual income level of people with dementia, but this is impractical in a simple survey. Instead the profile seeks to identify whether the person with dementia receives the basic level of state provision, which some may not, and whether this is supplemented by disability-related state benefits or private income.

Housing is probably the easiest indicator to use, serving both as an excellent indicator of other resources and as an important resource in its own right. Housing tenure denotes both security and control over the property. The distinction between owner-occupiers and others is important, partly as an indicator of other resources, and partly because owner-occupiers are deemed to have capital when it comes to paying fees for residential care.

As indicators of house condition the profile uses the presence or absence of certain amenities, on the basis that those houses which lack these amenities are generally those in worse physical condition, and the respondent's assessment of whether the house needs major repairs. The main housing problems this approach does not identify are those of location and neighbourhood.

The needs of carers People with dementia often rely upon the efforts of informal carers to maintain their existence in a domiciliary setting, but this can be at considerable cost to carers' own wellbeing.[17] A needs assessment must, therefore, take the needs of carers as well as people with dementia into account.

There are three components to be considered here: the actual involvement of the carer, which is important not just as an aspect of need but also as a response to the needs of the person with dementia; the practical or 'objective' impact on the carer's life and activities; and the emotional or 'subjective' impact on the carer and on their relationship with the person with dementia.[18] These factors represent needs in themselves; they can also be seen as important predictors of the availability of support for people with dementia.

The practical impact of caring is largely a consequence of time pressure[19] and of the inability to timetable 'supervision' in the same way as physical care.[20] The involvement of carers is gauged in terms of the profile's standard categories of need, which serves two purposes. On one hand, it gives information about the situation of the carer; on the other, it also provides information which is relevant for an assessment of the needs of people with dementia, as to whether their needs are met.

The pressures of caring are much more subjective:

> In the main a reward or problem [of caring] is anything perceived as such and it does not follow directly from the caring activity or behaviour.[21]

We experienced almost as much difficulty in designing questions on carer problems as we did with behaviour, and for a similar reason: that we initially attempted to encompass too much detail of the origins and processes of carer problems - the sort of information essential for the assessment of an individual case - rather than focusing on the outcome as perceived by the informal carer (or the professional respondent's view of the perceptions of the informal carer). The very substantial literature on the pressures experienced by carers of people with dementia gave no shortage of avenues to explore, unproductively. Eventually we resolved the problem by taking three simple questions to cover the carer's perception of practical problems arising from caring, emotional upset, and an overall carer judgement of coping.

The consideration of the pressure and stress on carers calls for a reflection on an element which is not directly considered within the profile, which is the emotional distress experienced by people with dementia. There are three main reasons for not including it. The first is that whereas emotional distress itself is very difficult to gauge, factors which lead to emotional distress (including loss of faculty and social isolation) are already taken into account. Second, emotional distress does not demand a direct service response distinct from other responses; it would do so only if there was a specialised service of this kind. The third is that the attempt to communicate with people with dementia about emotional distress may itself prove distressing, and this would be difficult to justify on an ethical basis. This relates to questions considered later in the chapter on ethical issues.

Discussion

The outline of the profile described here does not cover all the details required to make it fully operational; those are considered in more detail in chapter 8. What is important at this stage is the principle of the matrix approach, and its application to the circumstances of people with dementia. The matrix provides core information on:

- the need for services to compensate for deficits in activities of daily living and social functioning, and
- the need for services to moderate the impact of dementia upon family

carers.
The main exception to this relates to the need for diagnosis and direct clinicial treatment of cognitive impairment. The need for diagnosis is directly related to incidence, which can be derived from appropriate national studies. The main purpose of clinical treatment at present is optimisation of a patient's condition, rather than cure, which means that the need for clinical treatment is a direct function of prevalence.

It might be asked why it was felt necessary to develop a new profile when Bond and Carstairs had already developed one. The answer relates back to the purpose behind the Tayside Profile: the aim was to develop a brief tool suitable for collecting a minimum data set for analysis for planning purposes. Bond and Carstairs' scale was not suitable for this purpose.

> One of the [Bond and Carstairs'] schedule's drawbacks is that by virtue of its comprehensiveness, eliciting all the information required on dependency would prove a relatively lengthy process. It would be difficult, therefore, to envisage using the Clackmannan model to carry out rapid assessments of clients currently receiving residential or domiciliary services as a basis for planning decisions. ... managers would be unlikely to have the time or resources to undertake something as sophisticated as this.[22]

The Tayside Profile is much more economical in its approach. It aims to be no more than sufficiently comprehensive for the planning task. The Profile reflects the complexity and variability of the needs and circumstances of people with dementia[23] and carers in a way useful to planners, but it does so in a relatively simple format.

Table 4.1 summarises the essential components of the Profile.

Table 4.1
Tayside Profile for Dementia Planning

Dimension	Classification
Mobility	Independent Long interval Short interval Critical interval
Personal care	Independent Long interval Short interval Critical interval Personal care problems at night
Domestic tasks	Independent Long interval Short interval
Behaviour	Independent Long interval Short interval Critical interval Behaviour problems at night
Solitude	Living alone Time spent alone during day
Material needs	Housing tenure House condition Income
Informal carer involvement	Independent Long interval Short interval Critical interval Involvement at night
Informal carer problems	Coping Practical problems Emotional upset

5 Fieldwork method

The study was developed recursively; the process of testing and experimenting led to progressive refinement of the instrument. The first phase of the project was conducted in Perth, identifying the range of needs through interviews with carers and discussions with professionals. The results of this process are incorporated into the material in the preceding chapter. The second stage conducted a census of people with dementia in Angus district, which provided the basis for detailed analysis and experimentation with different approaches to the data which was collected. The third stage was a full field trial in Dundee. The basic process which was followed in each field trial consisted of

- a census of people with dementia, which provided a sampling frame for the application of the instrument, and
- collecting information about the sample, including extensive testing of the instrument in different contexts and methods of application.

The fieldwork design

In the chapter on planning, we argued that an instrument for planning purposes needs to provide information on individuals and on an aggregate population. There is an argument for avoiding individual assessment, and basing figures not on local surveys but on estimates based on national figures; the practice is widespread in the formation of community care plans. If a range of services is provided from which this range of needs can be met, the precise numbers which need to be provided may not be important. The advantages of this approach are twofold. First, it is administratively simple, and relatively costless; it requires no local fieldwork. Second, even if it is a compromise, it is not an unreasonable one. All figures are unreliable; national figures are not really very much worse, and may be better than a unrepresentative local sample. Jorm et al., in a secondary analysis of the literature on prevalence, found that although estimates of prevalence vary with definitions and populations, there was a consistent trend for prevalence to vary with age, with the prevalence doubling every 5.1 years.[1] The trend is confirmed by the figures from EURODEM.[2] Drawing on the rationale behind the use of indicators, this suggests that national prevalence figures can at least be used as a consistent benchmark against which services can be planned.

There are, however, disadvantages. Many of the nationally based figures are of questionable validity; there are substantial variations in the figures.[3] There may be large variations in needs locally; this is particularly true where services for elderly people, like residential care, attract a higher proportion of people with dementia into a particular locality. Last, and most important for the purposes of local planning, the relationship of national figures to planning issues is limited. National figures give some idea of inputs and needs for aggregate populations, but they do not necessarily explain their relationship, and it is difficult from aggregate figures of this type to see whether needs are unmet, or if domiciliary care might be substituted for residential care.

This kind of relationship can most effectively be identified by developing categories of need which can be identified for individual cases and then aggregated for the population as a whole. This does not mean, however, that every individual has to be assessed; it is possible to use a sample survey and subsequently to approximate for the total. Sampling is for the most part cheaper and quicker than a comprehensive procedure, and statistically speaking, random sampling is less likely to suffer from the systematic distortions associated with comprehensive assessments. The main disadvantage of sampling is that both the numerators and the denominators in the equation are uncertain; the effect of multiplying up from base figures can be to distort existing patterns. In a multi-agency, area-wide study there may be little alternative to sampling, though an existing area-based service may have another option, which is routinely to require all members of staff to make returns and so to acquire a fairly comprehensive set of data on its own clients.

The reasons for sampling in the course of this study were straightforward enough. This was a research project, and there were not the resources to collect data on everyone. We were looking only for indicators, and there was no added value in collecting fuller data. We were also concerned to test the instrument in a range of different settings, and to use different methods, which meant that a sample had to be arranged to meet those criteria. The same considerations would probably not apply to planners who wished to apply this process in practice; there is no problem in principle with seeking to incorporate the collection of data into the normal patterns of assessment, aggregating information from a range of sources.

There are two main options for the construction of a sampling frame. The first is to assess the whole population, or at least a large sample, which could be random or geographically clustered.[4] The sampling frame is the elderly population at large, from which the subset with dementia has to be identified and then carers and supporters. This is time-consuming and expensive. The advantage is that it identifies people not known to services.

The second option is to identify people with dementia from information held by services who might have contact with people with dementia and their carers.[5] The advantages of this procedure are:

- all cases which have presented or are likely to present demand in the short term will have been taken into account.
- the effect of assessing each and every case is of itself likely to affect the services' subsequent pattern of response
- The method does not disturb large numbers of non-dementing elderly people and carers who would otherwise have to be screened to find the small proportion with dementia.
- it is relatively cheap; much of the work is office-based (rather than the extensive fieldwork required with the screening approach)

The disadvantages are:

- It relies strongly on the motivation of service providers to supply the information: if there is insufficient cooperation, the method collapses.
- It will omit people not known to services, which might vary from area to area. The pattern of cases reported tends to reflect the existing demand for services. The effect of a comprehensive assessment can be to reinforce such trends.

We opted for the second approach. The arguments are not conclusive, however, and as part of the process of developing the Tayside profile we have tried to examine the implications of different approaches, so that the effects of different methods of estimation and approximation can be identified. This will make it possible for informed choices to be made subsequently depending on the context in which the instrument is to be used.

The procedure is described fully in chapter 7. The basic method was to identify people known to services by asking as many services as possible who they knew about, and cross-referring information from different services to eliminate possible double-counting. Once information had been collected about the whole population, it was possible to draw a sample and to compile profiles of that sample. We drew information from a range of respondents, and developed instruments in order to collect the information more effectively. There were, by the end of this process, two different instruments for collecting information. One, aimed mainly at professional staff, asked staff to make a judgment about the levels of dependency within the main categories of the instrument, with guidance notes about the process. Specific forms were designed for use in different settings, including community care, residential units and hospitals. The second, aimed principally at informal carers, used closed questions in simple language in order to acquire information about the level of dependency. These instruments were tested in a variety of situations; the material on that process is included in chapter 9.

Fieldwork: a summary

The field work which was undertaken is briefly described here. Later sections have fuller discussions of the process of identifying people for the census and the process of testing the instruments in practice.

The initial field trial

The first census of people with dementia aged 65 years and over was held in the Angus area on 1st November, 1992. The community sample list was obtained by requesting lists of people believed to be dementing from all major services (e.g. GP's, community nurses, home-help organisers, social workers, day care). Referrers were asked to supply the names and addresses of people with dementia and an informal carer (if known). The institutional sample was obtained by asking officers-in-charge, charge nurses, etc. for a list of people with dementia. Both psychogeriatric and geriatric 'routes' into care were covered. These lists were consolidated into a single master list from which samples were drawn. 857 people with dementia were identified, of whom 568 were resident in institutions and 291 resident in the community. This compares with an expected 1013 based on EURODEM prevalence rates. After allowing for cross-boundary flow to institutions, it was estimated that the true identification rate was 80% (809/1013). Of the estimated total 1063 people in dementia (including cross-boundary flow): 26% were in hospital, 27% in residential or nursing homes, 27% in the community and known to services (often the GP), and 19% in the community and not known to services (or, at least, not returned by them in the census). The most important group in identifying people with dementia in the community were general practitioners, who knew 58% of them.

This census provided the sample frame for the trials of various approaches. 498 assessments were made of 355 people (Table 5.1). Methods of administering the assessment were tested in residential and community settings, with validatory interviews. This stage was used to identify the advantages and disadvantages of different forms of administration of the assessment instruments, and to revise and refine the assessment forms.

Full field trial

This took place in Dundee, after the completion of the Angus stage. It began, as in Angus, with a census of people with dementia, as of 1st November 1993. 1,426 sufferers were identified, compared with the EURODEM estimate of 1,907. A further 178 were estimated to be known to non-responding services. The remainder may be unknown to services; men and younger people with dementia seem less likely to be known to services. Allowing for the non-response, and assuming those unknown were resident in the community, 55% of the 1,907 people with dementia were resident in the community, 19% in in-patient care, 10% in nursing homes and 16% in residential care.

The second stage in Dundee consisted of the administration of the assessment instruments to samples of carers of people living in the community and in institutions. Service personnel were involved in this phase. In order to test the robustness and ease of use of the instrument, we brought in a sizeable number of workers each administering a small number of interviews. 624 assessments were made of 450 people (see Table 5.1). The involvement of a wider range of professionals and informal carers gave the opportunity to examine the acceptability, reliability and robustness of the procedure in a variety of settings.

The Angus sample was intended to be, and was, broadly representative within place of residence strata. The Dundee sample set out to ensure that an adequate sample was obtained to test the reliability of the instrument. Maximising the numbers in the various categories, especially those poorly represented from the Angus phase, was the primary objective; no attempt was made to have a sample that was representative of Dundee. This meant in practice that many of those with no informal carer were not sampled since an objective was to increase the number with assessments by both an informal carers and a professional worker.

Table 5.1
Summary data: census, sampling and assessment

Outcome		Tayside		Angus		Dundee	
		N	%	N	%	N	%
CENSUS		2238	100	857	100	1381	100
NOT SELECTED							
Not sampled		621		229		392	
No approach, no carer		212		10		202	
Unable to sample		38		9		29	
OPERATIONAL SAMPLE		1367	100	609	100	758	100
CHANGED SITUATION							
Dead		157	11.5	90	14.8	67	8.8
Moved -	to hospital	78	5.7	38	6.2	40	5.3
	to RH	73	5.3	37	6.1	36	4.7
	to NH	39	2.9	17	2.8	22	2.9
	from area	5	0.4	4	0.7	1	0.1
	discharged	2	0.1	0	0	2	0.3
OTHER LOSSES		14	1.0	0	0	14	1.8
AVAILABLE FOR ASSESSMENT			(73.1)		(69.4)		(76.0)
REFUSALS							
Service refusal		114	8.3	39	6.4	75	9.9
Informal carer refusal		43	3.1	13	2.1	30	4.0
EXCLUSIONS							
Not dementing		23	1.7	15	2.5	8	1.1
Other		14	1.0	1	0.2	13	1.7
ASSESSED		805	58.9	355	58.4	450	59.4
NUMBER OF ASSESSMENTS		1122		498		624	

6 The local context of the surveys

Surveys of needs have to be set in the context of local demography, socioeconomic circumstances, and service levels. This chapter does that for the surveys in Angus and Dundee by comparing selected statistical indicators with Scottish average figures. This section is based upon a range of statistical sources.[1] The intention of the comparisons made here is to highlight major differences between the study areas and the Scottish average so as, first, to indicate if differences in survey results might stem from differences between study areas and, second, to illustrate that decisions on action to meet needs might vary depending on the characteristics of the area in question.

Data have been drawn from a number of sources and for a variety of dates within the period 1990 to 1992.[2] The Scottish average has been used as a reference point and comparison is therefore restricted to data which is available at national and local level. A comprehensive analysis would use a wider range of data and pursue at least some topics in greater depth.

Demography

Both rural Angus, with 16.7% of its population aged 65 and over, and urban Dundee (16.4% aged 65+) have relatively elderly populations compared with the Scottish average (15.1%) (Table 6.1).

Translating age structure into an estimate of the number of people with dementia requires the selection of a prevalence rate. The wide variation in prevalence rates reported by different studies is very well known.[3] There are many contentious methodological issues.[4] Much of the difficulty lies with marginal or 'mild' dementia.[5] This often involves a level of impairment which does not markedly interfere with normal daily functioning, and scores below the threshold in cognitive tests.[6] Low scores can also be explained by a low

Table 6.1
Age structure, 1993

	Angus	Dundee	Scotland
Total population	97,420	170,120	5,120,200
% population, age:			
65-74	9.3	9.7	8.8
75-84	5.6	5.2	4.9
85+	1.8	1.6	1.4

educational level, low socio-economic status, impaired physical health, deafness, other psychiatric illness or other factors affecting performance on tests which are unconnected with the presence or absence of dementia.[7]

There are numerous dementia prevalence studies in the literature, and an several syntheses have been published.[8] The prevalence rates from the meta-analysis by Jorm, Korten and Henderson[9] have been widely used to make local estimates but the more recent synthesis by the EURODEM group[10] has a number of advantages. EURODEM used more explicit and rigorous criteria for including or excluding studies. In particular it excluded studies which omitted institutional populations. Contrary to Jorm's assertion that the inclusion or exclusion of institutional populations makes little difference, it can have a substantial impact on the numerator in a prevalence calculation.[11] EURODEM also presents results for a wider spread of age groups and for the sexes separately, and provides data which can be used to calculate confidence limits.

In use, EURODEM appears to provide a mid-range estimate, a little higher than Jorm, Korten and Henderson but lower than other studies used by planners such as Bond and Carstairs.[12] In a study which screened all those aged 75+ in a Tayside town, the number of probable people with dementia identified was, after making a pro rata allowance for non-response, virtually identical to an estimate based on EURODEM.[13]

Applying the EURODEM rates to the mid-1993 populations for Angus and Dundee gives an estimate of 1,207 people with dementia aged 65 and over in Angus (95% confidence interval 950-1502) and 1,931 in Dundee (95% confidence interval 1515-2417) (Table 6.2). There is little knowledge of the extent to which prevalence varies by locality,[14] though the close fit between a EURODEM-based estimate and Carr's fieldwork results in a Tayside town suggests that EURODEM is an appropriate starting point in Tayside.

Local figures can be distorted by the presence of large institutional populations.[15] For example, it is known that there is some inflow of elderly people into longstay care in Angus, including about 30 psychogeriatric continuing care patients from Dundee.

Table 6.2
Dementia estimates, 1993

	Angus			Dundee			Angus & Dundee excl. Carnoustie
	Male	Fem	M+F	Male	Fem	M+F	M+F
65-69	46	29	75	88	53	141	208
70-74	87	94	181	147	170	317	478
75-79	55	129	184	92	211	303	466
80-84	101	217	318	145	348	493	775
85-89	61	212	273	81	342	423	666
90+	34	142	176	39	215	254	410
Total	384	822	1207	591	1340	1931	3003
Confidence limits (95%)							
Lower	*274*	*676*	*950*	*417*	*1098*	*1515*	-
Higher	*516*	*986*	*1502*	*803*	*1614*	*2417*	-

Socioeconomic characteristics

On a comparison of housing and economic indicators, Dundee city generally emerges as poorer than the Scottish average, while Angus, with a rural and small town settlement pattern, is either close to the average or better than it. For example, Dundee has a lower level of owner-occupation, fewer households with central heating, more households without a car and greater unemployment. Dundee does have a better than average level of w.c.'s and baths, but the number of households lacking such amenities is very small and increasingly concentrated in rural areas. The greater level of car ownership in Angus needs to be qualified by the greater necessity of a car in rural areas.

A relatively high proportion of the Angus population aged 75 and over is resident in longstay medical and social care establishments; in Dundee the proportion is only slightly higher than the Scottish average. The proportions of households containing persons of pensionable age and pensioners living alone show little variation. Angus has a markedly lower proportion of residents in private households aged 75 and over with a (self-reported) limiting long term illness. This may be a consequence of the higher proportion of this age group which is resident in longstay care establishments in Angus. A lower proportion of Angus households contain a dependant of pensionable age - that is, a person of pensionable age with a limiting long term illness - whereas the proportion in Dundee is relatively high. Details are given in table 6.3.

Table 6.3
Social indicators, 1991

%	Angus	Dundee
75+ resident in medical & care establishments	13	11
Households with persons of pension age	35	34
Pensioner households with lone resident	49	51
75+ in private households with limiting long term illness	42	49
Households with dependant of pensionable age	10	13

Services

Both Angus and Dundee have a high level of provision of specialist accommodation for elderly people (Table 6.4). The main variation is in the level of residential home provision. There is some cross-boundary flow from Dundee to establishments in Angus and there may also be some wider 'retirement migration' to establishments in rural areas. Dundee also has a markedly high level of provision of sheltered housing.

The level of provision of domiciliary services varies by service and District (Table 6.5). In both Angus and Dundee district nursing has lower than average coverage but higher than average intensity, with an overall above-average level of provision. Home help coverage is about average in Angus but the level of resources (measured by full time equivalent home helps) is low. Home help coverage is high in Dundee but with resources no greater than average. The implication is that intensity of service is low in both areas. The provision of day services is below average in both areas with the exception is psychogeriatric day care in Dundee. Meals-on-wheels coverage in both areas is average. Local data for community psychiatric nursing and social worker clients shows Angus to have lower service levels than Dundee.

Table 6.4
Specialist accommodation, c.1992

Beds per 1000 population over 75	Angus	Dundee	Scotland
Sheltered housing *(Dwellings/1000 pop 65+)*	51	150	41
Residential home			
- Social Work Department	39	39	29
- Voluntary	7	24	13
- Private	51	17	12
Nursing home	39	30	35
Geriatric continuing care	27	20	26
Psychogeriatric	26	22	20
Total	189	152	135

Table 6.5
Domiciliary and day services, c.1992

	Angus	Dundee	Scotland
District nurse visits			
- 1st visits age 75+/1000 pop 75+	265	279	304
- Visits per patient age 75+	42	35	28
Home help clients/1000			
- 65-74	37	57	41
- 75+	177	242	178
Home helps (full time equivalent)/ 1000 pop 65+	10	14	14
Day hospital places /1000 pop 75+			
- Geriatric	2.1	2.5	3.5
- Psychogeriatric	1.1	4.2	3.0
Day care places per 1000 pop 75+	20	9	23
Persons attending day care/ 1000 pop 75+	37	22	48

Conclusion

In summary, Angus and Dundee have more elderly populations than the Scottish average. Both Angus and Dundee have a high level of institutional provision, especially in Angus, though some of this may be accounted for by movements between districts. The implication of the data on institutional, domiciliary and day services is that, at the time of our fieldwork, elderly people with dementia in both Angus and Dundee faced a service environment with a resource bias towards institutional forms of care.

The demographic, socioeconomic and service characteristics of an area provide a context both for the interpretation of the results of surveys of needs and for the development of plans to meet the needs identified. In practice, more information has to be used, including qualitative information on local consumer and professional views.

7 A service-based census

A census provides, in principle, a useful basis for the construction of indicators about a population; as such, the results of the census procedure are important in themselves, and not only as a sampling frame for the later work. The fluctuating population means, of necessity, that results can never be precise, and it is important to treat what follows with some caution; even so, the censuses offer an important insight into the relationship between the prevalence of dementia and the delivery of services.

Method

The rationale for drawing on material from services was outlined in chapter 5. The Angus and Dundee censuses were conducted separately but did not differ in any material respects and can be used as one to describe the process.

In theory a census is undertaken on a single, specified day: in both Angus and Dundee we used 1st November. In practice, returns to the census (as with any survey) can take months to come in. Waiting for returns creates complications for the next, survey, stage if sampling is delayed until the last achievable responses have been obtained. A long delay at this point can lead to serious attrition of the sample frame, which the census is intended to create. It is difficult, however, to sample earlier, for example by taking a predetermined proportion of returns for each setting, since responses cannot be predicted and a wrong 'guess' could lead to under- or over-sampling in a particular setting.

The full range of services likely to deal with people with dementia was approached; the services are listed in table 7.2. Motivating service providers to participate in the census was crucial to the success of the method. Preparing the ground required negotiation and dicussion with managers and workers in health, social and housing services in the public, voluntary and private sectors. This took considerable time, but it was fundamental to the success of the censuses, and so of the whole study: if service providers do not see the process as worthwhile, it will founder.

Different census forms were used for institutional and for community services. The information collected was necessarily fuller for community residents (Table 7.1). As census forms were returned the information was crosschecked to identify people for whom more than one return is received. Individuals were then entered into a database as either a new record or as an extension of an existing record. Once complete, this database, subdivided by setting, forms the sample frame for the survey stage, which is described in a later chapter.

Table 7.1
Data captured by census forms

Community census form	Institutional census form
Service & worker making return Name Address Date of Birth Sex Carer name, address, telephone number	Institution making return Name Date of birth Sex

Identifying the population with dementia

A deliberately broad definition was used for the population of interest. In Tayside the definition given was:

> People aged 65 and over with a gradual loss of ability to carry out everyday functions because of failing memory, possibly coupled with personality changes and physical problems.

In a separate study in Forth Valley the definition used was:

> People aged 65 and over with problems of memory/confusion (as is caused by dementia).

Equivalent returns were obtained with these different definitions, suggesting that the target group is defined equally well in respondents' minds by either definition.

We have assumed that the population defined by this process approximates to the population with dementia. No clinical assessment of mental impairment was undertaken. For the purposes of providing most services - the main exception is clinical intervention itself - the clinical diagnosis of dementia is not necessarily crucial; what is important is the presenting pattern of need.

Identifying carers

Although the primary target population is people with dementia-like impairments, it was also important to identify informal carers, for two main reasons. First, some of the needs which have to be met are needs of carers, rather than of people with dementia. Second, the primary informants about many people with dementia will be their carers.

Few samples of carers are representative.[1] This is sometimes deliberate: a researcher may decide to study only carers who meet certain criteria, such as coresidence or visiting more than twice a week.[2] Often, however, the bias comes with the use of a particular sampling frame, most notably in studies recruiting by self-selection or using samples from carer organisations and groups. Another significant source of bias can be refusals: Wright had a 34% refusal rate, with refusal more likely from males, those working and those who may themselves be mentally disturbed.[3] There are other studies where it is not clear why the carer sample was much smaller than the elderly sample: for example, Charlesworth et al. interviewed 157 carers from a starting sample of 255 old people referred to geriatric, psychiatric or social services.[4] In many of the studies cited above the bias of the sample has been towards the 'heavy end' of caring, but this need not invariably be the case. Those feeling most overwhelmed by caring may be unable to find time to respond to research requests.[5]

One source of bias which has attracted criticism is that many studies have approached subjects through their pre-existing contact with services.[6] This may lead to samples of carers with lower tolerance and greater psychiatric morbidity, especially if the services in question are targeted on relieving such problems.[7] The method for the Tayside Profile is also service-based. The involvement of all relevant services in the census should minimise such bias, though it cannot eliminate it.

Not every person with dementia living in the community will have an informal carer. The figures differ widely; different studies have found 5%,[8] 18%[9] and 20-26%[10] of people with dementia to have no informal carers. It is still true that most people with dementia will have either an informal carer or one or more paid carers, such as a home help. In the Stirling University study, Carr found that 8% of the prospective sample (12/158) had neither formal nor informal carers.

In our study, we found that data about carers returned on our census form was not always reliable, and when we proposed to interview carers the data needed to be validated. Because the field trials included some assessments based only on the responses of service professionals, carer data was not always checked. Also, in the Dundee phase a large number without a carer recorded at the census were not pursued (see table 5.1): it is possible that a follow-up could have identified carers for some of these subjects.

The response of the services

All sources of census returns, in Angus and Dundee combined, are shown in Table 7.2. Staff in medical and care establishments, GPs, sheltered housing wardens, home helps, social workers, home helps and community nurses were the most important sources of referrals. GPs and sheltered housing wardens were particularly important sources of 'sole referrals' - that is, subjects referred by one source only - in the community. Seventy per cent of the 2238 persons were identified by only one service respondent. The particular results for Tayside reflect the pattern of services in the area, for example the distinctively high level of sheltered housing, and the differing level of enthusiasm of different services and individual workers for participating in the census.

Non-response by mainstream services in Angus was trivial - two small residential homes. The main non-respondents in Angus were small voluntary organisations. This is unlikely to have much impact upon the total number of individuals identified since the returns made by voluntary groups that did participate identified very few people who are not also identified by other services. Non-response in Dundee was more serious, with GPs in 55% of general practices and consultants responsible for 24% of geriatric continuing care beds not participating in the census. For a further 18% of geriatric continuing care beds only the total number of people with dementia was provided, without any identifying or demographic data. Lack of participation by a significant number of main sources can seriously weaken the census phase. Pro rata estimates of numbers can be made, provided a sufficient number of workers in a service participate and provided the proportion of participating workers is known. However, the individuals are lost to the sample frame.

It is clear from the table that the participation of both health and social services is necessary for a census to succeed, especially in the community, where health service returns in Tayside accounted for 44% of sole community returns while social services (including sheltered housing wardens) accounted for 53%.

Table 7.2
Census returns by referring source

*column percentage***

	All returns		Community residents	
	Total	Sole source	Total	Sole source
Community health				
GP	26.3	16.2	31.8	25.8
District nurse	6.7	2.3	13.0	5.7
Continence adviser	5.7	2.9	4.3	1.9
Chiropody	4.7	3.1	7.4	6.4
Day hospital	4.2	1.2	8.9	2.7
Health visitor	1.1	0.5	2.4	1.1
Comm. psy. nurse	1.1	0.3	2.2	0.8
Community social				
Sheltered housing	11.1	10.3	26.6	25.6
Home help	9.5	5.6	23.1	13.9
Social worker	9.5	5.2	14.9	8.4
Day care*	4.0	1.8	9.1	4.5
Occupational therapy	1.8	0.7	2.5	0.5
Voluntary/carer groups	3.8	0.8	6.2	1.3
Medical & care establishments				
Residential home	18.8	16.1	0.1	0.2
Psychiatric	13.7	14.6	0.2	0
Geriatric	11.1	12.3	1.5	1.3
Nursing home	6.7	5.2	0	0
Physiotherapy	2.7	0.7	0	0
Base N (=100%)	2238	1563	917	628

* includes voluntary day care

** percentages sum to more than 100% because of individuals being referred by more than one service.

How accurate is a service-based census?

Two types of error are possible in a census (Table 7.3).

- The inclusion of people who do not have dementia (over-enumeration).
- The omission of people who have dementia (under-enumeration).

Table 7.3
Types of error in censuses

	Dementing	**Not dementing**	
Returned in census	Correctly enumerated	Over-enumeration	Total returned in census
Not returned in census	Under-enumeration	Correctly not enumerated	
	Total with dementia		

Over-enumeration

Inevitably, some people returned in the census do not have dementia. To enable an assessment of the level of false positive returns, Levin's brief rating scale was completed by those making survey assessments.[11] This is based on six questions about memory and orientation (see Chapter 8). It has a score ranging from 0 to 6, with higher scores indicating greater impairment of memory and orientation, and was found by Levin to correlate well with psychiatric diagnosis. A score of under 2, without a diagnosis of dementia stated, was taken as indicative of a low probability of dementia. In addition, there were some cases where assessment did not proceed as a result of information obtained from a professional or carer which indicated that there was no dementia. To ensure no unnecessary upset, a denial of dementia by a carer was always taken at face value. People with dementia or possible dementia were not themselves approached. The ethical issues are discussed in chapter 11.

Levin scale ratings were made for most community residents assessed and for around 60% of institutional residents. Scores were not calculated for assessments in which there was missing data for any of the six questions. There were 551 subjects for whom there was a rating (Table 7.4). When weighted to reflect the censused population by place of residence, an estimated

11.9% (267/2238: 95% ci 9.5%-14.3%) of those returned to the census lacked confirming evidence of cognitive impairment. The 16% of community residents who were false positives is comparable with Levin et al.'s study[12] where 22% of those identified by services as confused were assessed by research psychiatrists as having no evidence of dementia.

Table 7.4
Subjects lacking confirmation of cognitive impairment by place of residence

Residence	Census total	Excluded before assessment	Total assessed	Assessments with Levin score		Total estimated lacking impairment*	
				Total	Score <2	No.	% of census
Mainstream housing	538	15	213	161	18	98	18.2
Sheltered housing	379	6	126	100	9	52	13.8
Residential home - LA	254	1	111	66	15	60	23.6
Residential home - private	249	0	90	49	7	36	14.3
Nursing home	247	1	106	78	6	21	8.6
Psychiatric hospital	313	0	103	53	0	0	0
Geriatric hospital	258	0	93	44	0	0	0
Total	2238	23	842	551	55	267	11.9

* weighted to census

The proportion of total referrals by different services in the Tayside censuses which were estimated to lack confirming evidence of cognitive impairment ranged from nil to 25% (Table 7.5). As might be expected, the most accurate identification came from hospital inpatient sources. The services with the highest proportion lacking confirmation of cognitive impairment were day care and residential home, followed by day hospital and home help. The result for day hospital might reflect the use of provisional diagnoses during assessment. It must be noted, of course, that the exclusion criteria used, especially the Levin scale, are not comparable with either the gold standard of psychiatric diagnosis or with standardised tests administered directly to subjects.

Table 7.5
False positives amongst census returns by referring source

	Total returns (number)	% estimated to lack confirmation of cognitive impairment
Community health		
GP	589	11
District nurse	151	13
Continence adviser	128	7
Chiropody	106	11
Day hospital	94	17
Health visitor	24	-
Comm. psy. nurse	24	-
Community social		
Sheltered housing	249	13
Home help	213	16
Social worker	213	9
Day care*	89	25
Occupational therapy	41	-
Voluntary/carer groups	85	7
Medical & care establishments		
Residential home	420	23
Psychiatric	306	0
Geriatric	249	0
Nursing home	154	11
Physiotherapy	60	0

* includes voluntary day care
\- not calculated where denominator <50

Under-enumeration

By definition, a service-based census can only identify those cases already known to services. On the basis of the EURODEM estimates, this seems to exclude around one third of all people with dementia and around one half of those in the community.

To assess the characteristics of those missed by a census it is necessary to have data from a simultaneous population screening survey and service census. Such a survey was undertaken by the Dementia Services Development Centre of Stirling University in 1991, covering the population aged 75 and over in a town in Tayside. The total number of people with dementia identified by screening, after pro rata uprating for non-response, corresponded very closely to an estimate for the town based on EURODEM prevalence rates. An anonymised data file was made available to the present authors for reanalysis, showing who was identified by screening but not by services.[13]

Before considering this data, it may be helpful to compare the number and demographic profile of people with dementia identified in Tayside with the expected number and demographic profile based on EURODEM. It seems younger people with dementia and men are not fully covered. (There was also a higher-than-expected number in the oldest age group. This may reflect some mistaken identification of dementia, particularly likely with frail very elderly people who may have sensory problems or depression.) It may be that people who were omitted from the census had a milder degree of dementia, so that they did not need services to be involved, or simply that the services had not yet recognised their needs. It is also possible that carers (especially spouses) might be 'shielding' them from service involvement. Both of these issues are more likely in the younger elderly age groups.[14] There may also be an understandable reluctance in non-health services, such as home helps or housing wardens, to identify cases without validation by medical diagnosis. Again, this would lead to greater omission of people with milder cognitive impairment.

Of 76 'sufferers' in the community in the Stirling University study, exactly half had been identified by the service census and half only identified by population screening (based on a score on the Mini Mental State Examination[15] of less than 25). Of 51 'sufferers' in residential care, 33 had been identified by the census and 18 only by screening.

People not identified by the service census may be less cognitively impaired. This hypothesis is supported by the Stirling University data, using Levin scale scores (Table 7.6). In the community, 37% of those identified by the service census and 84% of those identified only by screening scored <2 on the Levin scale ($p<.01$). In residential homes the proportions were 24% and 78%, respectively ($p<.01$). The same pattern, and level of statistical significance, was found on Greene et al.'s[16] behaviour and mood disturbance scale and, for those with informal carer respondents, on Jorm and Jacomb's[17] informant questionnaire on cognitive decline.

A second hypothesis is that people in private households who are not

Table 7.6
Levin Scores, Stirling University study, persons aged over 75

number

Levin score	Households		Residential homes	
	census (N=38)	screening (N=38)	census (N=33)	screening (N=18)
0	9	25	5	10
1	5	7	3	4
2	2	2	6	0
3	6	2	2	2
4	6	2	0	0
5	4	0	9	1
6	6	0	8	1
Mean score	2.8	0.6	3.5	1.2

identified by the service census would be more likely to have informal carers shielding them. This is consistent with the data, though the difference in the proportion with a coresident carer is not statistically significant: 24% of those not identified had a coresident carer compared with 10% of those identified (p>.05). The interviewed carer was a spouse for 21% (not identified) compared with 8% (identified); for 37% a child compared with 21%; and for 29% a formal carer compared with 58% (p<.01 for the last comparison).

The interviews in the Stirling University study were terminated after the questions on cognitive impairment if the Levin score was zero. Together with the effect of missing data for specific questions, this means that the number of subjects with 'needs' data is very small. Nonetheless, some indication can be obtained of the likely impact on estimates of needs of the omission of those not identified by a service census.

On a list of 14 mobility, housecare and selfcare tasks, a higher proportion of subjects identified in the census was impaired than of those not identified. Typically, for community residents, around twice the proportion of those identified by services was impaired compared with those not identified. The difference was much less in residential care. Those identified by services were also significantly more likely to have urinary or faecal incontinence (p<.05 for community and for residential).

Those identified in the census received more services in the month prior to interview than did those not identified by the census. This was particularly evident in the community sample, where the mean number of services received by those censused was significantly higher (2.6 vs 1.3).

Those identified in the census caused more stress to their carers, with only two out of ten self-reporting that they were coping 'well' compared with four out of six of those not identified by services ($p<.05$). Six out of ten carers identified by services wanted more service help, compared with one out of five of those not identified ($p<.05$).

Despite the small number of subjects with 'needs' data, these results consistently support the position that those omitted from a service census have considerably lower needs than those identified by a census.

In summary, those not identified by a service census are likely to have the following characteristics compared with those identified:

- less cognitive impairment;
- less physical impairment, or impaired performance of tasks;
- more commonly an involved informal carer;
- lower service use; and
- less carer burden.

The results of the censuses

The Tayside censuses obtained 3,195 returns, identifying 2,238 individuals. The data on carers were insufficient to make a precise estimate; they suggest that, overall, around one in five of community residents with dementia might lack an informal carer.

Although the censuses have evident limitations, they provide important indicators of issues where information was not otherwise available - about the proportion of people with dementia who are known to services, and the kind of setting people with dementia live in locally.

Who is known to services?

Completing table 7.3 with the results of the Tayside censuses shows that 66% of the estimated number of people with dementia (1971/3003) were identified as individuals by the censuses.

To estimate the total number of people with dementia known to services, an allowance has to be made for non-response. An estimate was made of the number of referrals not made to the census because of known non-response by services (N=211). This figure will include some people who would have little evidence of cognitive impairment (estimated N=19),[18] giving a net estimate of 192 known to services but not included in the census. Adding this to the 1,971 correctly returned in the census gives an estimate of 72% (2,163/3,003) of people with dementia being known by services as having problems of

Table 7.7
Identification of people with dementia in the censuses

	Dementing	Not dementing	Census total
Returned in census	1971	267	2238
Not returned in census	1032	-	
Dementia total (EURODEM)	3003		

memory or dementia. Exactly half (840/1,680) of those in the community with dementia were not known to services. A proportion of those not known may in fact be known to services for reasons of physical rather than mental frailty.

The proportion of people with dementia known to services in Tayside was rather lower than has been found in some other surveys. For example, Livingston, Thomas and Graham,[19] in a study concerned particularly with dementia and depression, found that few dependent elderly people were not in contact with services. O'Connor, Pollitt, Brook, Reiss[20] found that 86% of people with severe dementia, 62% of moderate and 49% of mild living in the community - 58% overall - were known to at least one of the following services: home help, meals-on-wheels, district nurse, day centre. Note that this list excludes GPs. Levin et al. found that GPs identified people with less severe dementia,[21] though they also found that GPs identified an average of 3.5 people with dementia per practice when 20-30 had been expected.[22] The literature as a whole is inconclusive on the extent to which GPs know of dementia sufferers on their lists.[23]

It is not clear if the difference between these surveys and that in Tayside is because:

- services in Tayside know fewer people with dementia than other services elsewhere
- services in Tayside do not recognise that the people they are in contact with have dementia, or
- the method, despite the adjustments made, understates services' knowledge.

It is of interest to compare the censuses in the two areas, though the results must be used with caution because only a small number of Angus institutional residents had Levin scales completed (Table 7.8). The results are very similar for the two areas.

Table 7.8
Comparison of census results in Angus and Dundee

	Angus		Dundee	
EURODEM estimate (%)	1071	(100)	1931	(100)
Census total individuals identified	857		1381	
Estimated non-dementing in census	125		160	
Estimated dementing in census (%)	732	(68)	1221	(63)
Estimated dementing known to non-responding services	3		189	
Estimated total known to services (%)	735	(69)	1410	(73)

Where do people with dementia live?

This is shown for Tayside in Table 7.9. This builds upon the analysis of enumeration errors by allocating the shortfall between the EURODEM estimate and the estimated total number of people with dementia known to services to the setting of ordinary housing in the community. A high response rate from most institutions, as was achieved in Tayside, means that their estimated total, after exclusion of the estimated number lacking evidence of cognitive impairment, is lower than the census figure. The allocation of all those unknown to services into ordinary housing as their place of residence is deliberately intended to be conservative. People in institutional settings whose dementia is not known are nonetheless receiving some care. People in the same situation in the community may be receiving no care of any kind. It is therefore more important not to underestimate the number of people in the latter circumstance than in the former.

As can be seen, over 40% of people with dementia are resident in institutions of various types. This is in contradiction to Jacques' view that '... there can be few places in the world where the majority, or even a large minority of dementia sufferers are in institutions.'[24] Regrettably, Kay's[25] pioneering study in Newcastle, now 30 years old, is still sometimes cited in support of the view that only a small minority, even of people with severe dementia, are in institutional care.

A wide range of prevalence of dementia has been reported from different institutional settings: 33-75% of residential home residents, 40-70% of nursing home patients, 70-90% of geriatric longstay patients and 80-90% of longstay psychogeriatric patients.[26] Tayside Regional Council estimate that between

Table 7.9
Actual and estimated place of residence of people with dementia

	Estimated total		Individuals returned in census	
	N	%	N	%
Ordinary housing	1339	46	538	24
Sheltered housing	341	11	379	17
Residential home - local authority	199	7	254	11
Residential home - private/voluntary	227	8	249	11
Nursing home	236	8	247	11
Psychogeriatric beds	314	10	313	14
Geriatric beds	347	12	258	12
Total	3003	100	2238	100

Table 7.10
Residents with dementia-like impairment as percentage of beds

	Angus	Dundee	Total	(Base N†)
Sheltered housing*	7	7	7	(5041)
Residential home - local authority	24	28	28	(715)
Residential home - private/voluntary	25	25	26	(865)
Nursing home	24	48	37	(636)
Long-stay geriatric	64	93	80	(434)
Psychogeriatric	85	60	70	(447)

* as % of dwellings

† denominator data refers to various time periods and is drawn from local statistical reports, particularly the Tayside Regional Council Community Care Plan

33% and 50% of residential home residents suffered from 'a marked degree of confusion'.[27] These appear to be over-estimates compared with the results of the field trials. We have figures only for the numbers of dementia residents as a proportion of beds, usually at the end of March five months after the census date (Table 7.10); this understates the prevalence. It would be more accurate to express prevalence as a proportion of residents at the time of census, but we do not know how many residents there were on that date. The unexpectedly lower level in psychogeriatric beds may partly reflect problems in establishing the denominator, and partly the application of a stricter definition of dementia in the most specialist service.

It seems, even taking these issues into account, that there do appear to be generally low levels of prevalence in non-hospital settings in Tayside when compared with the literature. This might be a consequence of the high level of institutional provision locally.

Discussion

Use of a service-based census to identify people with problems of memory or confusion is open to criticism on grounds of incompleteness and inaccuracy.

- It can never be more complete than is the coverage of the target population by services. It is, however, valuable to be able to obtain a local estimate of what that coverage might be.
- It is vulnerable to total or partial non-response by services, though an estimate of the loss to the census from partial non-response can be made for the main services.
- It is vulnerable to an unknown amount of unsystematic non-response because of the reliance placed upon individual workers' ability to identify people in the target group on their caseload. Some workers will systematically review casenotes to do this, others will rely upon memory.
- In some cases names may be withheld because of ethical concerns or, where carer consent has been sought at the census stage, because of refusal of carer consent. This might introduce a systematic bias. For example, one voluntary organisation received consent to pass over only 19 out of 50 possible names. (Many of the missing names might have been returned to the census by other sources.)
- The census does not apply any strict diagnostic test of 'dementia'. Although allowance can be made by excluding those who fail to show sufficient evidence of cognitive impairment, this does not mean that the rest of the census population has dementia. The informant-based screening undertaken is necessarily crude since it has to be quickly

and easily administered. The checking undertaken should, however, serve to exclude those least likely to have dementia-like problems. The point must be emphasised that the census is intended to be of people with dementia-like problems. For needs assessment at a population level this is satisfactory; it would not be appropriate at an individual level, or for a clinical study.

- The process of taking a census introduces a systematic bias into the assessment of needs. The census is taken as of a particular day, but returns do not come in till later. Because dementia is progressive, this means that people's situation is likely to be worse by the time the assessments are made, and this is not counterbalanced either by individuals whose need may have lessened or by people with milder dementia coming into the population being studied. There is a tendency, then, to over-estimate the needs of the whole population, which is independent of the question of identification of people with dementia.
- The census is cheap to conduct. A census requires 2 months whole-time equivalent research assistant time spread over a period of about 4-5 months. Including salary, travel, stationery and postage gives a total revenue cost of £2,500-£3,000 for an area with a population of around 250,000. Accommodation and equipment costs would be extra.

Given the relative simplicity of the method compared with population screening of a large sample, the return of an estimated 66% of people with dementia in the census, after excluding apparently inappropriate returns, appears satisfactory. The return of 50% of people with dementia in the community is less satisfactory, but the finding is not out of line with the level of service knowledge suggested by the literature. As expected, the method fails to identify many people with mild dementia in the community - those not known to services or not recognised by services.

8 Administering the profile in practice

Chapter 4 described the profile in outline. When it came to applying the concepts in practice, it was necessary to specify the constituent elements of the matrix more precisely, and to devise methods by which the material could be compiled and returned. A large part of our activity in the fieldwork was concerned with refining and testing different approaches and issues; the technical data from those tests are presented in the following chapter. In this chapter, we will consider the issue of operationalisation - how a concept and approach can be translated into a practical instrument.

Preparing to collect material in different settings

Because people were identified in different places, the kind of information we were able to ask for varied according to the setting where they were placed. For professionals, the kinds of questions which were asked were general and open. We offered the broad categories with a note of explanation on the form, and added notes of guidance. Ample space was given for comment. For informal carers, the approach was necessarily different. A series of closed questions were asked, framed in simple language. Questions offering alternatives were separated into their constituent elements. (The form for carers is, in consequence, rather longer than the forms for professionals.)

The basic settings we identified were:

- in hospital care,
- in residential care and nursing homes, and
- in the community (including supported housing).

Questions which applied in the community would not necessarily apply in other settings. Information about informal carers and financial circumstances were not appropriate to hospital or residential care. Questions about solitude were inappropriate for people living in a group. No questions about services were asked for hospital residents. The effect of these differences was, of course, that the forms used for residential care were considerably shorter than those used for community care, and the forms for people resident in hospital were shorter still.

At the same time, there were still questions which proved difficult to answer in certain settings. Questions about domestic tasks often had to be answered hypothetically in an institutional setting. For example, all residents may be checked routinely at night whether they have a 'night need' or not. Some respondents from institutions felt unable to answer these questions. However, if it is not possible to ascertain what people's functional capacity is, it is also not possible to establish whether they are appropriately placed or served; omitting the questions would simply lose the data. It is worth noting that there is a case for expanding institutional profiles still further, so as to obtain community data for patents in 'longstay' hospital or residential/nursing homes who might subsequently be considered for discharge.

Any data collection form evolves from its basic form into a final product. In the development of the profile there were twenty different field tested versions of the four different formats of the profile, as well as innumerable in-house versions and one-off pilots. They included:

- Three versions of the questionnaire for informal carers.
- Five versions of the form for completion by community professionals.
- Five versions of the residential/nursing home form.
- Two versions of the hospital form.

The final versions, which are reproduced in the appendices, therefore draw upon a long process of improvement and refinement. Some of this process is common to any questionnaire; for example, the simplification of format, questions and language to be understandable by respondents. Other parts of the process reflected the subject matter and the difficulties of capturing unambiguously the key elements of need for people with dementia and their informal carers.

Arranging interviews

We decided, for ethical and practical reasons, to concentrate on returns from third parties - mainly professionals and carers. The practical arguments are straightforward: obtaining information from people with dementia would require difficult and sensitive fieldwork, considerable resources and cross-validation, with uncertain success. The ethical arguments, which are complex, are considered in greater detail in chapter 11. Any profile or index based on the observations and perceptions of third parties requires both knowledge of the situation and judgement as to the needs revealed in the situation. Completion of the Tayside Profile therefore requires knowledge of the person with dementia and carers, and it also requires judgement. Those closest to the person with dementia - such as informal carers - are likely to have the best knowledge, but their own needs may colour judgments about the needs of the person with dementia, and in any case their judgement is likely to differ from that of professionals. There is no simple resolution of this problem, and as we shall see in the following chapters it has implications for the reproducibility of results when different informants are used.

Prior to making contact with any sampled informal carer in the community, permission for this had been sought from the most involved professional. This also enabled confirmation that the sampled person was still living, that the identified carer was still involved, and that there were no circumstances (e.g. carer illness or family dispute) which might make an approach inappropriate. If permission was forthcoming, then the informal carer was contacted by telephone or letter, depending on the preference expressed by the professional, and given an explicit choice of participation or non-participation on the clear understanding that either choice would have no effect on the services they or the person they were caring for received.

The information to be collected

The information which we had to collect was of two kinds. The first was, of course, the information necessary to the construction of the profile, relating both to needs and available resources. Beyond this, though, it was necessary to compile further data which could make it possible to relate the sample to the whole population - consideration of identifiers, demographic details, and settings - as well as some measure of cognitive impairment. It would be possible to add other data, such as ethnicity, which might have greater relevance in other locations. However, care must be taken not to overload the profile with peripheral data of limited use and value in the context where it is applied.

The demographics of people with dementia The questionnaire and the forms contain information to identify the person with dementia and the carer or other respondent, together with their addresses or a longstay establishment name. Date of birth and sex are asked to confirm the data recorded in the census, or to replace missing data since not all census returns contain dates of birth.

Place of residence is a key dimension for analysis and (if necessary) for weighting of sample results to be representative of the total known population with dementia. Longstay establishments and extra-care (very sheltered) housing can be identified and classified from service lists but this is not always possible for 'ordinary' sheltered housing. The term 'sheltered housing' is often used loosely to refer to a wide range of types of housing, some of which is little different from mainstream housing with a remote communication device. Sheltered housing was identified, for the purposes of the trials, as housing with a warden.

Details of informal carers Recording basic demographic data about informal carers proved unexpectedly difficult, because both informal carers and professional workers sometimes included paid staff, particularly home helps, as 'informal carers'. The definition and textual emphases minimised this, though there were still some instances of misrecording. Errors can, however, be identified easily from the response to the question on the relationship of the carer to the person being helped.

This section also contains a question on whether the recorded carers themselves have a wider network of support. This enables the identification of single-handed unsupported carers, a group in whom service planners might have a particular interest.

Evidence of cognitive impairment It cannot be assumed that people with dementia will be correctly identified by service respondents. In circumstances where assessment of the (possibly) dementing individual is not feasible or appropriate, informant reports drawing upon the knowledge of informal carers or closely involved professionals have been found to be a reliable way to screen out people without dementia,[1] though in our experience there can be misleading reports, often based on denial (especially in early dementia) or on fear of the person with dementia being 'taken away'.[2]

Levin et al. used a six-question 'screen' with informants.[3] The questions are:

1. Does the person you help or care for often forget the names of family or friends seen regularly?
2. Do they often lose track of what is being said in the middle of a conversation?
3. Do they often get confused about what time of day it is?
4. Do they often get confused about where they are?
5. Do they have difficulty working out how to do ordinary everyday tasks?
6. Do they often have difficulty remembering recent events?

Dementia is improbable if less than two problems are endorsed. In Levin's study mean scores 'were strongly associated with the psychiatrists' diagnoses of dementia and its degree',[4] though the extent to which it classified individuals correctly is not reported. The instrument used in Tayside incorporated a brief checklist based on Levin's screening questions.

Our surveys in Angus showed Levin's checklist to be as efficient at identifying people who probably did not have dementia as a checklist based on the longer 11-item Intellectual Functioning Scale of the OPCS Surveys of Disability.[5] Of 153 assessments, 12 had a Levin score of less than 2 and no known diagnosis of dementia, compared with 10 with an OPCS score of less than 3. The OPCS scale was not used in the Dundee fieldwork.

The Levin checklist, like the OPCS checklist, is basically about memory-related abilities and cannot exclude memory impairment from causes other than dementia. The diagnosis is often not known by informal carers, and may not be available to others. The particular purpose of asking about the diagnosis is to ensure that no inappropriate diagnosis is known to the carer (e.g. depression, epilepsy, head trauma, learning disability). Questions on time of onset and whether the condition was worsening over time were tested but found to add no further material information. It must be emphasised that the quesstions used do not provide any clinical validation that the appropriate population is included in the survey, but their use does ensure that the surveyed population has intellectual impairment and no known alternative diagnosis.

There are three main reservations about using a screening device of this kind. The first is that it reduces estimates of overall demand in a way which may not be reflected in practice. The very fact that people thought to have a cognitive impairment have been returned in a service census indicates that someone in a service has thought it appropriate to return them, and this may be a truer statement of the demand for services. Second, dementia is a fluctuating condition, and particularly difficult to identify in its early stages. A rapid test for dementia-like conditions is likely to throw up false negatives - people whose mental state is lucid at the time of enquiry, or whose social functioning is adequate in a particular context. Third, the tests are approximations; they work in aggregate because false negatives are likely to be balanced by false positives. If people are selected for inclusion by services who have usually known them for a time, it is not necessarily the referring services who are mistaken.

Screening was important for this project, for two reasons. First, the procedure was being tested for applicability to people with dementia-like conditions, and it was basic to establishing validity that it should be seen to apply to people with dementia. Second, it was based on a sample, and there needed to be some way of relating the circumstances of the sample to the whole population. There may be circumstances - for example, where the profile is compiled through routine information gathering by a service - where this kind of screening is not thought appropriate.

Identifying people for assessment

The numbers of people interviewed are listed in chapter 5. 2,238 people were returned in the censuses. 805 of these were assessed at least once, with a total of 1,122 assessments being completed. A response rate of just under 60% was achieved in both Angus and Dundee, with the main losses arising from death and removal of the subject.

A higher service refusal rate was experienced in Dundee - 13% of those eligible, compared with 9% in Angus. This was largely because more professionals in Dundee were asked to complete forms themselves; it was not because of more refusals of permission to approach carers. Refusals of permission to approach carers included both examples of carers under extreme stress and cases where the relative of an individual with early dementia was unaware of the problem. Among informal carers a higher refusal rate was experienced for husbands (30%) and sons (24%) than for wives (18%) or daughters (11%).

Nearly one quarter of losses in the community were due to removal of respondents, almost all of which was into institutional care (Table 8.1). Refusals were at an acceptable level (18%) but the compounding of losses and refusals meant that only 46% of those sampled in the community were in fact assessed. Levin's survey, which used a similar method, achieved an almost identical rate: 150 interviews from 319 approaches to carers (47%).[6] Response rates from institutional settings were dependent upon death and removal rates. Removal almost always meant transfer to another institution.

Table 8.1
Sampling for assessments by place of residence

	Community	Residential	Nursing	Psychiatric	Geriatric
Operational sample (N); %	(673) 100	(245) 100	(146) 100	(161) 100	(142) 100
Dead Moved Other losses	7 23 1	9 7 1	11 2 3	24 10 0	23 6 0
Service refusal Carer refusal	12 6	1 0	12 0	2 0	5 1
Exclusion	5	1	1	0	0
Assessed %; (N)	46 (306)	81 (198)	72 (105)	64 (103)	66 (93)

The higher refusal rate for nursing homes arose from the refusal of one multi-home company to participate in the assessment stage.

There is inevitably a time delay between the nominal census date and assessment. As Table 8.2 shows, effort put into shortening this time is well repaid by a reduction in losses due to mortality and removal. Elderly people with dementia are not a static population: dying and moving from community to residential or hospital care are common.[7] Levin et al. followed up 410 people with dementia identified by services. After an interval of 6-12 months only 59% were still at home: 21% were dead and 20% in institutional care.[8] They also mention problems of sample attrition caused by interviewing not beginning until six months after their service census.

Table 8.2
Impact of delay to assessment upon mortality and removal losses

	Angus	Dundee	Forth Valley
Mean delay (days)	231	123	70
% operational sample lost by death/change of location	31%	22%	12%

Several factors contributed to the slow achievement of assessments in Angus and, to a lesser extent, in Dundee. Some of these are avoidable.

- The timing of the research involved a census date of 1st November in Angus and Dundee. There is inevitably delay over the Xmas/Hogmanay period and a date avoiding main holiday periods is preferable. A period of two months or so is necessary to obtain and consolidate all the census returns, regardless of the time of year.
- Until all census returns are returned, sampling cannot take place. (Though sampling can be broken down by setting and proceed as full returns for each setting are obtained.) The longer it takes to achieve all census returns, the more subjects already returned will have died or moved.
- Obtaining permission to approach carers adds further delay. In Angus, permission was sought from *all* those who had referred an individual in the census before a carer (or professional informant) was approached. This was cumbersome as well as time-consuming. In Dundee only the 'most involved' professional's permission was sought.

- Interviewing takes time. In Angus, return of postal questionnaires took 118 days, whereas interviews were spread over 230 days. (Both of these figures relate to the first assessments, and not to re-interviews for reliability testing.)

Since the people with the greatest needs might be presumed to be the most likely to die or to move to a more intensive care setting, losses on a substantial scale because of delays between census and assessment could in principle result in an underestimate of needs. Because the circumstances of others in the cohort are deteriorating, people with more severe needs are replaced by others. The main category of people with dementia which is likely to be underestimated is, then, people with mild dementia, whose conditions may deteriorate but who are not replaced within the count.

Despite the losses, the demographic profile of the achieved sample in Angus, where a representative sample was intended, was remarkably similar to that of the censused population. The census had a mean age of 85.4 years compared with a mean age for the survey of 85.1 years. 78% of census returns were female compared with 77% of assessed survey subjects. There were no statistically significant differences between the census and survey results on age or sex by place of residence.

Collecting data for the profile

The kind of information which has to be collected for the profile, and the rationale for collecting it, was outlined in chapter 4. Some of the problems in operationalising the data stem from the complex nature of dementia itself. The ability of people with dementia is often variable from day to day and week to week. Individuals are allocated to needs categories based upon their 'current' ability but where this fluctuates over time, between different levels of need, the allocation is to the highest level of need (most frequent level of intervention) since it is this level for which carers and services must always be prepared. Behaviour-related needs are identified on the basis of current behaviour, which may be affected by medication taken by the person with dementia or by current therapy or stimulation which they are receiving.

There are problems which relate to the categories which are used: ambiguities have to be resolved, and patterns of classification have to be rendered consistent. The greatest problems relate to the identification of behaviour. It can be difficult to decide whether people's problems in mobility, personal care or the performance of domestic tasks reflect behaviours rather than dependency in relation to those dimensions. In general, if carers intervene to prevent inappropriate attempts at personal care or domestic tasks (e.g. turning a cooker on at random, or undressing during the day), this has different implications for service responses from the inability to perform such tasks, and it should be attributed to the behaviour dimension.

The third main issue is the place of personal judgment. We have tried to minimise the scope for judgements to differ by reducing as many elements of the profile as possible to a basic measurement of the frequency with which intervention is required for broad categories of need. The analysis of behaviour is still dependent on judgment: it is impossible to remove from informal carer reports the 'watchful waiting' that, for many, characterises their constant anxiety about what the person with dementia *might* do. To the extent that this reflects the person's need for observation to trigger preventive action, it is an appropriate indicator of level of need. However, it may overstate the level of attention actually needed. Conversely, it is possible that staff in specialist psychiatric hospital or nursing and residential home settings might be more tolerant of extremes of behaviour and understate needs.

Service receipt The range of services which might be used by people with dementia and carers, and the complexity of patterns of service, means that it is not feasible to relate service inputs closely to time intervals during the day. We opted to ask about the number of days in the last month during which the person with dementia had received services. This does not distinguish between short-interval and critical-interval support - that is, it does not identify where service is being provided intensively and more often than once a day in a person's home. This problem could be overcome by recording occasions of service contact rather than days but service receipt more than once a day was too rare in Tayside for us to test out this option.

A significant problem with dementia can be the refusal of people with dementia to accept services which are offered. This can add appreciably to the pressures on informal carers and hasten institutional admission. However, it also reduces demand for community services and so the level of need that has to be met. The profile records, for each service, whether it has been refused by the person with dementia.

The services included in this section of the profile need to be those available in the locality in which the profile is being used, and the locally appropriate names for services need to be used. Respite care, because it was generally provided within a time frame, was asked about through a different format, but it is possible for respite care to be provided regularly in different localities.

We found that informants were not always sure of which facilities were day *hospitals* and which were day *centres*. The informant can be asked to give the name of any of these facilities attended so that errors can be identified and service use correctly allocated.

Recording and processing the information

The forms were designed to allow the easy recording of information on computer. The forms used for professionals were compact (1, 2 or 4 sides) and featured

- all main entries in two columns
- separate space for entry of notes
- forced choices - there are no 'Don't know' options on the forms, though all contain sufficient space to enable professionals completing forms to write this in.

The informal carer questionnaire covered 8 sides, plus a blank page for notes. It used standard right-justified tick-boxes wherever possible, and also had forced choices.

Because we were undertaking extensive examination of the results, we used SPSS-PC for analysis.

The profile in summary

The dimensions of the instruments used in practice, with their component parts, are shown in Table 8.3; this expands on the basic model described in chapter 4. In summary, the profile consisted of two sections on demography (of the person with dementia and carers), one on cognitive screening, seven on needs (including carer problems), and two on informal and service support. The areas considered for the person with dementia are similar to the areas suggested by Marshall as desirable for the *individual* profiling of residents in long-term care.[9]

Table 8.3
Tayside Profile for Dementia Planning: operational form

Dimension	Components
Demographics	Age Sex Place of residence
Evidence of cognitive impairment	Levin's screening questions Known medical diagnosis
Mobility	
Personal care	Day, night
Domestic tasks	
Behaviour	Day, night
Solitude	Time spent alone during day Live alone/not
Material needs	Housing tenure House condition Income
Informal carer demographics	Number Coresidence Relationship Age Sex Informal support to carers
Informal carer involvement	Day, night
Informal carer problems	Coping Practical problems Emotional upset
Service receipt	Respite Domiciliary/day Service refusal by person with dementia

General points

This chapter has been concerned mainly with practical details - the nuts and bolts of how we went about what we did. For people who wish to use the methods we have developed in other settings, it is important to emphasise that what we were doing was a research project, and that context had implications for several of the decisions we made in the design of the fieldwork. For example:

- We chose to construct a sample because we had no practical alternative. Planners who are part of major services have the option to collate information as part of standard assessment procedures.
- We based the sample on a census taken at a particular date because we had no other way of determining the size and constitution of the population in the area. Planners may have the option of keeping a running tally, which avoids the bias in figures implied in using a fixed date. (There is however the potential for distortion if data are only collected during crises.)
- We used a checklist to confirm evidence of cognitive impairment because it was necessary to ensure that people had such problems if we were to test the validity and reliability of our instruments in the right context. The arguments for screening may be less relevant for a service in practice.
- We had to negotiate consent with professionals, which was a time-consuming process, but which had the advantage of improving compliance. It is difficult to generalise from this experience to anticipate the situation for routine use in other localities.

It follows from this that the circumstances in which the Profile may be used are likely to vary, and some of the procedures will accordingly be different. The rationale behind the Profile does not depend on it being applied through an exact mirror of the procedures we have adopted. It is intended to provide useful indicators, and these indicators can be obtained by different means. There is a risk, however, that varying the conditions can also change the quality of information obtained, and the next chapter discusses some of the effects that different procedures are likely to have.

9 Testing the instrument in use

A useful assessment instrument must be acceptable to those intended to use it and produce valid and reliable results. In this chapter we consider these aspects of the Tayside Profile. For those who plan to use the profile, it is important to mark out the main findings from the field trials.

1. Four main methods were used to collate information. These were
   - A community form was used as an interview record in the community with both informal and service informants, and for self-completion by service informants.
   - A carer questionnaire was used for self-completion by informal informants.
   - A residential/nursing home (RNH) form was used for self-completion by RNH workers.
   - A hospital form was used for self-completion by hospital staff.

Telephone interviews were attempted but proved to be an unsatisfactory way of obtaining information.

2. The reliability of using different methods of administration of the profile on the same respondents is generally satisfactory.

3. The collection of factual data by the profiles was reliable where the information was known to respondents, but not all our respondents did know basic information about people with dementia. Professionals often had limited information about some dimensions, especially the circumstances of carers.

4. Because the circumstances of people with dementia change rapidly, there are some problems in gauging reliability over time, though our results were satisfactory.

5. There are important differences in the judgments made by professionals and informal carers, and the decision to obtain information from one source rather than another can have a large effect on the data obtained.

This chapter examines the issues for each question in the Profile. The material is more technical than in the preceding chapters, but it is important for people who plan to use the method.

Acceptability

Acceptability is a largely qualitative issue, of whether respondents found the instrument easy and appropriate in use. However, there are also quantitative indicators which can give some indication of acceptability; for example, an unacceptable instrument is unlikely to achieve a high response rate, or individual questions which are seen as unacceptable or inappropriate might have high non-response rates.

Four assessments of acceptability were made:

- the views of service providers completing forms;
- the views of informal carers;
- response rate; and
- the level of missing data.

Views of Service Providers Fifteen service providers in Angus commented on the form. Fourteen made favourable comments, mostly along the lines that the form was easy to understand, clear and simple to complete. Some commented that it was comprehensive or covered the main issues. Nine respondents made negative comments. Four commented on the difficulty of providing clear-cut answers. Three commented on the difficulty of completing the form because of their own incomplete knowledge, which is not an issue of acceptability *per se*. Two commented on aspects of the form which were subsequently revised (print size and the need to note refusal of services). One felt that there should be a section asking if the client had other problems not identified by the form, though in practice such data would almost certainly not be usable for planning.

Nursing staff on two short term psychiatric and geriatric wards were asked to comment on an extended version of the hospital form, which included a section on community data for patients being considered for discharge. Favourable comments were the same as those expressed by community services. Negative comments related mostly to hospital staff's lack of knowledge of home circumstances and difficulty answering the 'community' section. In the main section of the hospital form, domestic tasks were considered irrelevant by some respondents.

Views of informal carers The views of informal carers were sought during the design of the postal questionnaire, with the design being modified to take account of issues and problems raised. No negative comments were subsequently made in the course of using the instrument with informal carers.

Response rate An instrument unacceptable to potential respondents is unlikely to achieve a high response rate. Response rates in the Tayside surveys were outlined in chapter 5. Refusal rates were low. Ignoring all reasons for non-response except for refusal gives an overall refusal rate of 16.3% (157 refusals out of 157 + 805 assessments). This probably overstates the level of direct refusal, since the willingness of services to co-operate with research was a major element in refusals: some community refusals came from services refusing access to carers, usually for reasons unconnected with the nature of the Profile, while others were services themselves refusing to respond. These were not distinguished in our statistics.

In the community, the ratio of refusals to people for whom assessments were completed was 1:2.4, but this includes refusals by professionals to allow access to carers. An alternative measure is that there were 42 informal carer refusals for 195 first assessments, a ratio of 1:4.6, which appears reasonable for this kind of enquiry. In institutional settings the refusal:assessment ratio varied from 1:66 in residential homes to 1:6.2 in nursing homes. A corporate nursing home organisation refused to take part in the assessment phase. Psychiatric and geriatric wards had ratios of 1:26 and 1:12, respectively.

Missing data A certain level of missing data is virtually unavoidable in any survey work, especially where forms or questionnaires are self-completed by respondents, but a high level of missing data can indicate that a question or item is poorly designed or perceived as inappropriate or unanswerable by respondents. The level of missing data varied by data item and type of respondent (Table 9.1).

The lowest level of missing data (15 items/100 assessments) was obtained when informal carers were interviewed. The second lowest level (77 items/100 assessments) was when informal carers completed a postal questionnaire. There was evidence of a 'learning effect' when people completed two questionnaires: people completing a first questionnaire had an omission rate of 94/100 assessments compared with an omission rate of 45/100 for later questionnaires. Minor changes to the questionnaire between use in Angus and Dundee did not reduce the overall omission rate (70/100 and 81/100, respectively). It is of note that a version used subsequently in Forth Valley, which had further minor changes from previous versions, had an omission rate of 150/100 assessments. This might be a better reflection of use *in vivo* than the research field trials.

Professionals are more accustomed to completing structured forms than are informal carers. The omission rate for professionals was therefore unexpectedly high: 106 items/100 assessments when interviewed, 135/100 assessments when self-completing the community form. However, the evidence is that omissions were because the data was unknown rather than that

Table 9.1
Missing data

Missing data as percentage of completed assessments

Respondent	*Informal carer*		*Professional worker*			
Administration and form	*Postal form*	*Interview with community form*	*Interview with community form*	*Self-completion community form*	*Self-completion residential/ nursing form*	*Self-completion hospital form*
Physical	3	2	0	1	1	0
Selfcare	4	1	0	1	1	0
Selfcare night	4	1	2	1	0	0
Domestic	8	0	0	1	24	19
Behaviour	6	1	0	3	<.5	0
Behaviour night	7	1	2	1	0	0
Main carer relationship	0	0	2	2	x	x
Main carer age	6	1	6	24	x	x
Main carer sex	1	0	2	3	x	x
Carer supported	11	2	6	12	x	x
Carer involvement	7	0	6	7	x	x
Carer involvement at night	2	0	6	9	x	x
Carer practical impact	3	1	16	15	x	x
Carer emotional impact	4	2	14	16	x	x
Carer coping	4	1	14	9	x	x
Solitude	2	0	8	2	x	x
House tenure	2	0	0	3	x	x
Housing quality	2	3	4	4	x	x
Income	2	2	16	22	18	x
BASE N (=100%)	169	130	49	148	335	197

x - item not applicable

the question was in some way unacceptable. Professionals did not necessarily know about informal carers or income. There was some evidence of a 'learning effect' on second completions but not nearly so marked as for informal carer postal questionnaires.

In residential and nursing homes and in hospitals missing data were a problem only in respect of domestic tasks, which a significant minority of respondents regarded as irrelevant, and income (in homes), which was unknown to some respondents.

Missing data are of crucial importance to the application of the instrument for planning purposes, and have to be minimised. This argues strongly for the use wherever possible of interview rather than self-completion forms, though the difference in the amount of data gained is much greater for interviews with informal carers than it is for professionals.

Telephone Interviews There was one other aspect of acceptability which we tested: whether carers could be interviewed over the telephone. In practical clinical work a telephone interview can sometimes be the only way of speaking to someone, and it can be useful though it is always very clearly inferior to a face-to-face interview. Both English and American studies have reported the use of the telephone for carer interviews,[1] and in survey work it has been commented that 'for most straightforward market research questions the telephone will give the same answers as a face to face interview.'[2] However, the Tayside Profile does not ask straightforward market research questions.

We approached the interviewing of carers over the telephone cautiously. When we found, after only a small number, that they appeared to cause greater stress both to respondents and to the research interviewers, whose stress was a direct reflection of the distress they felt was being caused to carers, we abandoned this method. Telephone interviews provide neither the privacy of a postal questionnaire nor the scope to establish rapport which a face-to-face interview offers.[3]

Validity

Validity refers to the extent to which an instrument measures what it is intended to measure. For the Tayside Profile this is the needs of people with dementia and their carers, at a level of generalisation appropriate to planning. In quantitative social research, validity is often tested against some form of 'gold standard': for example, the gold standard for mobility might be an personal assessment by an experienced physiotherapist. To provide such gold standards for all the components of the Profile for use with a general (dementing) population sample was beyond the scope of the Tayside project. Instead we asked the much simpler questions of whether the results of the instrument appeared valid to a range of professionals and, as part of the process of development of the instrument, whether results matched the expressed views of informal carers.

Validity was assessed qualitatively using the comments of informal carers during the development of the Profile, a diary exercise with a small number of carers, the comments of professionals completing forms, and a review of discrepancies between respondents' written comments and their choice of pre-coded answers on completed forms. We also experimented with interviews with people with dementia themselves.

Comments of informal carers Semi-structured interviews were undertaken with the carers of 25 people with dementia as part of the process of developing the Profile. In some cases information was also gathered from service professionals. All but two were living at home, though only three lived alone and 21 attended some form of day care or hospital, reflecting the main source for this convenience sample. The purpose of these interviews was to guide the development of the profile by identifying the important dimensions from the perspective of the carer, but of course we already had a list of what we considered to be relevant dimensions and the interviews provided validation of this.

The main dimensions already identified were supported by the results of these interviews. The importance of the emotional component emerged very clearly; it was given additional emphasis by 14 of the 25 carers being spouses.

Carer diary Five carers (of nine approached) completed daily diary sheets for one week (range 5-8 days). Each sheet recorded, in two-hourly blocks, any problems the person with dementia had, the assistance the carer provided, services or others visiting the house and whether the person attended a service outwith the house. The data in the diaries confirmed the research workers' previous ratings of carer involvement and problems. Again, the emotional component was particularly evident. Services correlated well with previous reports. Although this small scale exercise was a 'success', most of the carers found keeping a diary in this form an onerous and depressing task. This was in total contrast to the views expressed by those who had participated in the semi-structured interviews, which were generally perceived as a positive and rewarding experience.

Professionals' comments The views of service providers referred to in the previous section are relevant to validity in that they endorsed the dimensions included in the Profile. The only dimension not endorsed (by some) was the inclusion of domestic tasks on the long-stay hospital form, a point which has been discussed previously. No specific additional dimensions were identified for inclusion.

Evident discrepancies The pro-forma designs of the Profile included space for written notes alongside the precoded responses under each dimension. In addition, throughout the development and testing of the Profile we were concerned to identify discrepancies so that the question format and phrasing could be adjusted to eliminate them. The relevant issues have already been considered in chapters 4 and 8 and need not be repeated.

Interviews with people with dementia Although the ethical and practical arguments led us to seek information from third parties, we thought it important to experiment with a small number of interviews with people with dementia. There are two main justifications for wishing to do so. The first is to accept that the views of people with dementia are still important. People with dementia can make sensible statements about their needs, and express their opinions and feelings.[4] The second is practical: there are a number of people with dementia who are best placed to respond, because they have no informal carers, and whose contact with professionals may be limited at the point of assessment. At the same time, there are important reservations to make. One is ethical: people with dementia are especially vulnerable, and it is important to avoid contact which may cause unnecessary distress. The second is practical: it was important to validate the comments. For that reason the people with dementia who were selected were those who had formal or informal carers who could also answer about their circumstances.

The initial interviews showed a very marked tendency to underestimate needs by comparison with the assessment of carers or professionals. This observation is not unique to the circumstances of people with dementia, but it meant that it was inappropriate to pursue the issues further in the context of this research, which was to be a low-cost survey for planning purposes. One member of our team has since developed this work further.[5] The points of principle will be returned to later in the chapter on ethical issues.

Reliability

Reliability refers to the reproducibility of results. Different elements of reliability tested in the Tayside Profile were:

- test-retest reliability, administering the instrument twice in the same form to the same informant;
- inter-method reliability, administering the instrument twice to the same respondent but using a different method on each occasion; for example, self-completion on the first occasion (T_1) and an interview on the second occasion (T_2);
- inter-informant reliability, administering the instrument to different informants at T_1 and T_2, ideally using the same method though this was not possible where methods were intentionally designed differently for different types of informant.

Missing data, from unanswered questions in the assessment, also affect reliability.

Four basic methods and profile formats were used.

- The community form was used
  (a) as an interview record in the community with both informal and service informants and
  (b) for self-completion by service informants.
- The carer questionnaire was used for self-completion by informal informants.
- The residential/nursing home (RNH) form was used for self-completion by RNH workers. For testing purposes only it was also used an as interview record.
- The hospital form was used for self-completion by hospital staff. For testing purposes only it was also used as an interview record.

The complexity of testing the reliability of an instrument while also running a full scale field trial cannot be under-estimated. The length of time which elapsed between the initial (T_1) and follow-up (T_2) assessments (detailed in table 9.2) reflects the operational difficulties encountered. The longer this time, the more difficult it becomes to interpret results on reliability because the results obtained at T_2 may differ from T_1 because of a real change. This is all the more important with an unstable condition such as dementia, and the length of time elapsed in the Tayside Project was often longer than desirable.

For statistical reasons, explained below, a minimum number of 30 cases is desirable in each combination to be tested. While three of the combinations had a slight shortfall in numbers, there was initially a major shortfall for service worker self-completion of the community form at T_1 and T_2. To rectify this, an additional sample was taken after the conclusion of the main phase of fieldwork in Dundee to boost the number to 30.

Two measures were used to assess the level of agreement between T_1 and T_2 administrations of the instrument. The best test is the nonparametric Kappa coefficient which measures agreement taking into account the likelihood of chance levels of agreement.[6] Simple Kappa was used for 2x2 tables and weighted Kappa for larger tables.[7] Kappa has a range from 1.0 through 0 to -1.0. A Kappa of 1.0 indicates complete agreement between T_1 and T_2; 0 indicates a level of agreement no better than would be expected by chance; -1.0 indicates complete disagreement. A level of 0.6 or greater is usually regarded as satisfactory.[8] To allow for the effects of the long delay between T_1 and T_2, we have taken a level of 0.4 or greater as acceptable. Kappa requires a minimum of 20 cases for valid calculation for 3x3 tables and 30 for 4x4 tables.[9] Some comparison tables are 4x4 and one must be cautious about accepting the Kappa statistics as valid for these comparisons where the

Table 9.2
Reliability tests: number of cases and time between assessments by method/informant combinations

T_1 method; informant	T_2 method; informant	Mean time (days) T_1 to T_2	N cases
TEST-RETEST (same informant, same method)			
Interview; informal carer	Interview; informal carer		
Postal qre; informal carer	Postal qre; informal carer	21	31
Self-completion; worker	Self-completion; worker		
Self-completion; RNH	Self-completion; RNH	22	40
Self-completion; hospital	Self-completion; hospital	26	30
		44	30
		23	31
INTER-METHOD (same informant, different method)			
Postal qre; informal carer	Interview; informal carer	33	32
Self-completion; worker	Interview; worker		
Self-completion; RNH	Interview; RNH	50	28
Self-completion; hospital		36	31
	Interview; hospital		
		26	25
INTER-INFORMANT (different informant, varying method)			
Postal qre; informal	Self-completion; worker	37	28
Interview; informal carer	Self-completion; worker	49	38

comparison sample is fewer than 30 cases. A highly skewed distribution of responses, as was found for some of the Tayside data, makes it very unlikely that a high Kappa can be achieved since a high level of agreement can be obtained by chance with such a distribution. In such circumstances a simple measure of percentage agreement - the percentage of cases with the same response at T_1 and T_2 - is useful if one is simply interested in whether the overall patterns at T_1 and T_2 are similar.

A large number of comparisons are made in this chapter and the following criteria were applied to identify results which could be judged as acceptable.

- Kappa(w) ≥ 0.6 *and* agreement $\geq 70\%$ = good agreement.
- Kappa(w) $\geq 0.4 < 0.6$ *and* agreement $\geq 70\%$ = satisfactory agreement.
- Kappa(w) $\geq 0.4 < 0.6$ with agreement $< 70\%$ = moderate agreement.
- Kappa(w) not calculable *and* agreement $\geq 70\%$ = satisfactory

agreement.

- Kappa(w) < 0.4 = unsatisfactory agreement.

(Kappa is not calculable where the number of rows and columns in a comparison table are not equal or where the number of both rows and columns is one.)

Reliability: testing the components

The reliability of the individual components of the Tayside Profile can be divided into two sections, excluding the Levin questions on evidence of cognitive impairment which were not repeated: (1) factual components such as age, co-residence and use of services and (2) subjective assessments such as mobility, behaviour and carer problems.

Factual components

Those items regarded as factual are demographics of people with dementia, co-residence, material needs, informal carer demographics except for informal support to carers, and service receipt.

All assessments were compared with the data on age, sex and place of residence recorded at the census stage. Of 1,122 assessments, 1,053 (93.9%) agreed with the census on age at census date; 64 (5.7%) differed by one year, 3 differed by 2 years, and only 2 differed by a greater amount, one of which was identified as a wrong census age. There were no disagreements on subject's sex. There were 18 (1.6%) instances when the place of residence did not agree between the census and all assessments. The differences were all between mainstream housing and sheltered or other supported housing. (The census record was often based on housing lists, which may have been out of date or inaccurate.) Fifteen cases should have been listed as in sheltered or supported rather than mainstream housing, while three moved the opposite way.

Levels of agreement between T_1 and T_2 responses on coresidence and informal carer demographics are shown in Table 9.3. Test-retest results are good, except for the informal carer postal questionnaire result on co-residence which is satisfactory. Some spouses did not include themselves as coresidents in earlier versions of the questionnaire; this was remedied in later versions.

The reliability of using different methods of administration of the profile on the same respondents is good for all except three results. The unsatisfactory results for informal carer postal questionnaires, compared with interview for co-residence and for the number of carers, agaïn reflects spouses who failed

Table 9.3
Agreement on coresidence and carer demographics

	Co-residence		N carers		Carer relation-ship*		Carer age*		Carer sex*	
	%	K	%	K	%	K	%	K	%	K
SAME RESPONDENT, SAME METHOD										
Informal interview	100	1.	100	1.	100	1	100	1.	100	1.
Informal postal	80	.60	82	.77	98	.97	78	‡	95	.89
Worker self-completion	100	1.	84	.82	96	.95	92	‡	96	.92
SAME RESPONDENT, DIFFERENT METHOD										
Informal postal/interview	73	.45	67	.29	93	.90	82	‡	93	.71
Worker self/interview	100	1.	75	.66	100	1.	43	‡	100	1.
DIFFERENT RESPONDENT, DIFFERENT METHOD										
Informal post/Worker self	81	.62	41	.03	85	.80	50	‡	89	.76
Informal interview/ Worker self	92	.82	67	.33	89	‡	37	‡	83	.65

‡ Kappa not calculable
* Reliability tested on first-named carer

to identify themself as co-resident. The divergence between the age reported by professionals for carers at T_1 and T_2 possibly reflects professionals' overall lack of knowledge of carers. There was a large number of cases with no data (see Table 9.1) and where an age was given it was probably often a 'best guess', liable to vary slightly at a second attempt.

Comparison of data for the same situations but taken from different respondents using different methods produces an intriguing pattern of results. Coresidence, relationship of carers and sex of carers all showed good agreement. Number of carers and carer age showed unsatisfactory agreement. The latter probably reflects professionals' poor knowledge of ages. No explanation can be given for the differences on the number of carers.

Agreement on indicators of possible material need was good for test-retest and inter-method reliability on all three indicators and with all types of respondent (Table 9.4). However, agreement between informal carers and professionals was only moderate for tenure, and unsatisfactory for house condition and income sources. The latter reflects professionals' lack of knowledge of the incomes of people with dementia, where they hazarded any information - no data was given by professionals for over one fifth of cases. The difference in results for house condition reveals house condition to be a matter of judgement as well as fact. All professionals thought that the housing situation was satisfactory, but some informal carers did not share this view. This might also reflect the different format of the questions. Informal carers were asked specifically about inside sanitation, central heating and need for major repair; professionals, although guided to these factors, were asked to make a single overall judgement.

Data on service use is 'factual', but we could not test its reliability at individual level because of the likelihood of real changes having taken place in service use between T_1 and T_2. Service use by people with dementia is very susceptible to substantial change over quite short periods, and the mean time

Table 9.4
Agreement on material needs

	Tenure		House condition		Income sources	
	%	K	%	K	%	K
SAME RESPONDENT, SAME METHOD						
Informal interview	90	.80	97	.90	93	.88
Informal postal	95	.92	95	.83	87	.80
Worker self-completion	100	1.	95	.65	90	.84
SAME RESPONDENT, DIFFERENT METHOD						
Informal postal/Interview	97	.90	90	.77	74	.56
Worker self/Interview	89	.67	100	1.	67	.57
DIFFERENT RESPONDENT, DIFFERENT METHOD						
Informal postal/Worker self	74	.42	76	-.12	41	.03
Informal interview/Worker self	88	.57	80	‡	56	.31

‡ Kappa not calculable

between the T_1 and T_2 data was 3-7 weeks, depending on subgroup - more than sufficient time for services to change. By comparing aggregate patterns of service use, however, we were able to assess their similarity at T_1 and T_2 and so to gain some indication of the reliability of the data overall.

For most test groups and services the level of variation is within that which could be expected (Table 9.5). There were some wide variations but these were spread across services and groups and not clustered in a way which would cast suspicion on the reliability of data collected for a particular service, from a particular source or by a particular method.

In summary, the collection of factual data by the profiles (as modified in the light of early results) was reliable where the information was known to respondents. This is an important proviso given the variability of knowledge about carers demonstrated by professional respondents. Of the individual profile components, only house condition raises serious concern since its reliability appears to be affected by choice of respondent (which raises a question also of validity) and question format.

The assessment of need

Returns on the needs of people with dementia, carer involvement, support to carers and carer needs, depend to some degree on the judgment of the respondent. This does not mean that these factors cannot be assessed in terms of set criteria, but it does imply that responses are also dependent on personal perceptions. Data on the assessment of needs is shown in Tables 9.6-9.8.

Data on mobility is acceptable except when informal carer postal data is compared with professional self-completion data. In this comparison, informal carers were more likely to rate people with dementia as having no mobility needs (71%) compared with formal workers' ratings (57%).

Test-retest reliability for personal care is good except for night need in hospital. This is caused by the highly skewed distribution of such need: 90% at T_1 and 84% at T_2 were considered to require night assistance with personal care. Results for inter-method reliability are satisfactory for personal care in the daytime but more mixed for personal care at night, again being influenced by skew. Inter-informant reliability is unsatisfactory. However, for informal postal/worker self-completion the overall levels of need (i.e. the marginal totals - which is what would actually be taken as planning data from the Profile) are very similar at T_1 and T_2 even though individuals are rated very differently. This is not the case for informal interview/formal self-completion, where the former give an overall pattern of higher need.

Table 9.5
Percentage using services in past 28 days (past year for respite)

		GP	Community nurse	Social worker	Home help	Day sitter	Day hospital	Day centre	Respite care
SAME RESPONDENT, SAME METHOD									
Informal interview	T_1	29	32	13	48	13	16	32	36
	T_2	36	26	6	48	10	16	32	36
Informal postal	T_1	22	45	15	50	22	22	22	38
	T_2	20	45	15	42	22	25	15	38
Worker self-completion	T_1	37	43	37	60	7	40	13	33
	T_2	40	37	33	60	10	40	13	33
SAME RESPONDENT, DIFFERENT METHOD									
Informal postal/ interview	T_1	50	31	16	47	16	16	31	16
	T_2	41	28	9	50	16	6	28	16
Worker self completion/ interview	T_1	7	50	14	68	4	21	7	25
	T_2	21	50	18	78	4	25	36	28
DIFFERENT RESPONDENT, DIFFERENT METHOD									
Informal post/Worker self completion	T_1	29	25	21	46	39	32	43	50
	T_2	21	25	25	50	7	32	46	29
Informal interview/ Worker self completion	T_1	42	29	18	50	11	21	58	37
	T_2	29	29	13	47	5	16	47	39

Test-retest reliability for need for assistance with domestic tasks is satisfactory. Inter-method reliability is more mixed, though marginal totals are similar for T_1 and T_2. Likewise, the unsatisfactory inter-informant result for informal carer postal/formal worker self-completion is offset by similar marginal totals. This is not the case for informal interview/formal self-completion, where the former gives a substantially higher level of overall need: 84% short-interval compared with 60%.

Test-retest reliability for behaviour, both day and night, is shown in table 9.7. Although the assessment might seem particularly vulnerable to personal perceptions, the results are mostly acceptable. The unsatisfactory results for

Table 9.6
Agreement on the assessment of needs for mobility, personal care and domestic care

	Mobility		Personal care		Personal care - night		Domestic	
	%	K	%	K	%	K	%	K
SAME RESPONDENT, SAME METHOD								
Informal interview	97	.97	87	.89	90	.79	97	.87
Informal postal	82	.73	69	.71	100	1.	76	.59
Worker self-completion	77	.59	77	.77	97	.78	83	.73
RH/NH self-completion	73	.70	80	.82	83	.67	69	.50
Hospital self-completion	74	.63	84	.64	81	.15	100	1.
SAME RESPONDENT, DIFFERENT METHOD								
Informal postal/interview	56	.42	52	.56	81	.50	75	.33
Worker self completion/interview	82	.74	54	.56	89	.34	75	.51
RH/NH self completion/interview	80	.74	60	.53	77	.52	53	-.11
Hospital self completion/interview	88	.85	84	.69	80	.17	100	1.
DIFFERENT RESPONDENT, DIFFERENT METHOD								
Informal post/Worker self completion	44	.10	39	.27	82	.44	57	.11
Informal interview/Worker self completion	76	.67	34	.30	76	.08	67	.31

institutions are partly offset by marginal totals being similar at T_1 and T_2. However, hospital self-completion data is unsatisfactory with no consistency at either individual or aggregate levels. Following a familiar pattern, inter-method reliability is mixed but inter-respondent reliability is mostly unsatisfactory. These unsatisfactory results are not redeemed by any similarity of marginal totals. We described in the previous chapter the difficulty we had in developing this part of the Profile and undoubtedly some of this difficulty is reflected in these results, which combine data from several test versions of the Profile. There are too few cases in the Tayside data to analyse separately the different versions.

Table 9.7
Agreement on the assessment of behaviour

	Behaviour		Behaviour - night	
	%	K	%	K
SAME RESPONDENT, SAME METHOD				
Informal interview	74	.63	90	.61
Informal postal	73	.68	97	.92
Worker self-completion	62	.59	93	.81
RH/NH self-completion	70	.68	67	.32
Hospital self-completion	52	.05	68	.31
SAME RESPONDENT, DIFFERENT METHOD				
Informal postal/interview	52	.53	87	.68
Worker self completion/interview	54	.30	82	.19
RH/NH self completion/interview	42	.21	81	.56
Hospital self completion/interview	64	.53	52	.10
DIFFERENT RESPONDENT, DIFFERENT METHOD				
Informal post/Worker self completion	50	.30	71	.30
Informal interview/Worker self completion	50	.32	89	.65

All results for solitude are acceptable except for informal carer postal/formal worker self-completion (Table 9.8). Formal workers gave a higher solitude rating: no informal carers rated a person with dementia as isolated (alone more than 10 hours a day) compared with 19% so rated by formal workers. The question of whether informal carers feel they themselves have informal sources of support shows acceptable test-retest reliability (Table 9.8). Inter-method reliability is mixed, with informal postal/interview having an unsatisfactory result, though marginal totals are broadly similar for both methods. Inter-respondent reliability is unsatisfactory, though marginal totals are similar for informal interview/formal self-completion.

Carer involvement might be considered a matter of record, but the definition of 'involvement' is partly a matter of perception. Results, both for day and night, are acceptable with two exceptions (Table 9.9).

Table 9.8
Agreement on solitude of people with dementia; other informal support to carers

	Solitude		Support to carers	
	%	K	%	K
SAME RESPONDENT, SAME METHOD				
Informal interview	100	1.00	90	.80
Informal postal	82	.73	74	.41
Worker self-completion	83	.74	77	.55
SAME RESPONDENT, DIFFERENT METHOD				
Informal postal/ Worker self completion	75	.50	59	.07
Informal interview/ Worker self completion	94	.91	73	.45
DIFFERENT RESPONDENT, DIFFERENT METHOD				
Informal postal/ worker self completion	43	-.04	50	-.09
Informal interview/ worker self completion	82	.52	60	.17

Informal interview/worker self-completion produced higher estimates of daytime involvement from informal respondents than from formal workers for involvement more than once a day at regular times, with lower estimates for involvement only once a day, though apart from this there was considerable similarity in the marginal totals for both groups (with 58% and 64%, respectively, assessing involvement as critical interval). The other unsatisfactory result, for worker self-completion/worker interview in respect of involvement at night, had an unsatisfactory Kappa statistic. This was mainly a consequence of skewed data: most carers in this subsample were not involved at night.

The three indicators of carer needs all had similar patterns of reliability results and can be considered together (Table 9.9). Test-retest reliability was acceptable for all, as was inter-method reliability with the exception of worker self-completion/interview results for emotional upset. The marginal totals, however, were similar: respectively, 50% and 56% of carers were rated as experiencing emotional upset. All of the inter-respondent results for carer need

Table 9.9
Agreement on carer involvement and needs

	Carer involvement		Carer involvement - night		Practical problems		Emotional upset		Coping	
	%	K	%	K	%	K	%	K	%	K
SAME RESPONDENT, SAME METHOD										
Informal interview	77	.65	94	.86	90	.80	83	.63	90	.51
Informal postal	61	.49	77	.54	86	.70	94	.89	97	.84
Worker self-completion	88	.89	92	.83	95	.90	90	.81	96	.88
SAME RESPONDENT, DIFFERENT METHOD										
Informal postal/ interview	57	.42	73	.47	73	.43	81	.62	88	.51
Worker self completion/ interview	81	.81	78	.37	69	.43	69	.38	94	.76
DIFFERENT RESPONDENT, DIFFERENT METHOD										
Informal postal/ Worker self completion	50	.40	77	.54	56	.14	44	-.17	81	.24
Informal interview/ Worker self completion	61	.36	89	.76	50	.02	57	.07	73	-.06

were unsatisfactory. For emotional upset the marginal totals were similar, but for practical problems and coping there were systematic differences between informal and formal respondents: the latter were more likely to consider that there were practical problems and difficulty caring with coping. The informal carer respondents themselves were less likely to perceive practical problems and hardly any thought they were not coping with caring.

Reliability: discussion

A large number of comparisons were presented in the previous section. We made allowance for the time delay between T_1 and T_2 by adopting a relatively low threshold of 0.4 for Kappa. We made allowance for the fact that our interest is in aggregate data for planning purposes by looking at percentage agreement as well as Kappa, and by exploring the degree to which T_1 and T_2 aggregate totals were similar even when individual data differed. Even after this, there remain a number of unsatisfactory results. What might explain these?

The main possible reasons identified from qualitative review of the Tayside field trials for unsatisfactory test-retest reliability were:

- Real change in the person and situation being assessed. This includes continuing deterioration but also improvement, especially in relation to behaviour through, for example, appropriate drug therapy. The time delay between T_1 and T_2 assessments was more than ample for changes to have taken place in elderly people with dementia. For example, in hospital settings, there was evidence that some patients had a reduced need for day or night intervention regarding behaviour. This might be attributable to the impact of therapy, including drug treatment. It could alternatively reflect the lessening of behavioural difficulties through, for example, increased immobility or passivity but there was no evidence of this. In residential and nursing home settings there was evidence that increased passivity had an impact upon the T_2 assessments.
- Real change but with an over-reaction to this in the change of rating. This was suggested, for example, when Residential/Nursing Home staff noted that a resident's behaviour was now independent, compared with the previous critical interval, because he or she was 'content to sit'. In other words, they created no behavioural problems for staff and therefore were seen as having had no need for behaviour-related intervention.
- Some differences arose because of continuing refinement of the assessment instrument and associated definitions. This introduced some inconsistencies when a change was introduced or a definition clarified between T_1 and T_2 assessments. It also means that the overall comparison aggregates different, evolving, versions of the instrument for both T_1 and T_2.
- Errors in form completion. There were instances where one response was clearly inconsistent and likely to be a simple form-filling error.

But the main problems of reliability were not found in the simple test-retest situation. They were in the inter-method and, particularly, the inter-respondent results. What might explain these?

- Lack of knowledge of the complete situation was encountered with some services. This seemed particularly to be the case when the respondents came from a service, such as day care, which did not necessarily know of the full domestic situation, such as the level of involvement of carers. This can be exacerbated where the person with dementia presents different 'faces' in different situations.
- There were apparent differences of judgement or perception between respondents regarding the level of need. These were found mainly between informal carers on the one hand and workers (including the research interviewers, who were both qualified social workers) on the other. It is not possible to accept the judgement of one or other party as definitive. Informal carers may over-rate the need for assistance because of their concern for their relative or their own level of stress, but they may under-rate it because of being habituated to a situation. Professionals may be prone to under-rating need because of habituation to difficult situations. Bond and Carstairs obtained Kappa results, comparing elderly residents' own assessments and those of caring staff for individual components of dependency, equivalent to those reported here.[10]

In many cases review of the limited available data revealed no evident reason why the response should be different. The behaviour of the same lady could be described as: 'OK - plays dominoes at Centre and willing to be involved in what is going on', which would be rated as independent, and 'Inactive - needs stimulation, encouragement', which would be rated as critical interval dependency. There may be a substantial random element caused by the variability of dementia and of the emotions of those caring informally for people with dementia. Most reliability problems relate to areas, such as behaviour and carer emotional upset, which might be expected to have a considerable potential for day to day fluctuation and for differences in the perception of need.

In the absence of a definitive 'gold standard', when there are apparent differences of opinion there is no clear reason why one opinion should be preferred over another. It might be argued that workers in formal services are able to make a more realistic and objective assessment of need but our data does not allow this issue, which is essentially one of validity, to be determined. However, there were sometimes explicit problems of needs being assessed in a service-oriented framework, a problem also identified in community care needs assessments.[11] For example, one service respondent wrote: 'lives with his wife who is able to support him in a domestic situation' and categorised the subject's domestic support needs as nil when he was, in fact, incapable of performing any domestic tasks for himself. Furthermore, we found some tendency for both informal carers and home helps to rate the time intensity of needs as equivalent to their own current level of input. It was not always clear that this was an appropriate level, in the absence of corroboration from other data.

In summary, the reliability of the Profile is satisfactory - indeed, given the time delay between first and second assessments it is better than satisfactory. The problems identified through testing its reliability raise issues more of validity than of reliability - but validity by what criterion? Can we assume that professionals provide the most accurate and dispassionate assessments, or are informal carers, with their intimate but more emotionally-influenced knowledge, the better sources of information?

Conclusion

The difficulties of undertaking reliability testing within a large scale field trial with finite resources of time, money and people willing to complete repeated assessment forms are substantial. Although we managed to achieve close to the required numbers for most of the combinations of method and informant being tested, it proved extremely difficult to achieve a satisfactorily short gap between T_1 and T_2 assessments.

The time lag between T_1 and T_2 assessments adds difficulty to the interpretation of the reliability results. The natural short term variability in the population with dementia is very substantial. Individual symptoms are often not persistent and can affect individuals with differing intensity at different times. Early testing of the Scottish Health Resource Utilisation Groups (SHRUGs) on elderly longstay inpatients found that variables which were reasonably reliable on retesting after 1-2 days could not be demonstrated to be reliable with a time delay of two weeks to retesting because of real change in patients.[12] Brace and colleagues have observed that:

> standardised assessment forms may have limited use where older people have complex needs, being too crude to deal with the multiple changes and complexities of these situations. Assessments could be valid for one day only and in one context.[13]

Despite the time lag, test-retest results proved satisfactory. On this basis it does not much matter whether the respondent is an informal carer or a professional and how the profile is administered. If cost is no obstacle, interviewing informants achieves the most complete and reliable data, with the smallest amount of missing data. In Tayside the researchers undertaking the project interviews were qualified and experienced social workers. Their decision-making in their interviews with informal carers would often find common ground with other professionals, which might not always be an advantage.

There are differences in results depending on the method of administration, but realistically the choice of method of administering the Profile is likely to be decided on cost grounds. The main choice on this basis is between informal carer questionnaires and worker self-completion forms. There are swings and roundabouts here: the former has the more complete data overall, but some questions were more fully answered using the latter. Informal carers were better informed on demographic details and carer problems. The crucial questions about the needs of people with dementia themselves were answered more fully by professionals than by informal carers.

It is clear from the analysis in this chapter that different informants - informal carers and formal service workers - are likely to give different results. Without further research to identify which, if either taken as a group, provides the more valid view of the situation, the best approach is to ensure that any survey contains a mix of informants. (This applies to a community sample: in institutional care there is no realistic alternative to relying upon staff assessments.) Ideally one might seek to obtain information from the person with the best overall view of the situation, who will be an informal carer or a closely involved worker, most likely to be a domiciliary services worker or a care manager.

It is appropriate that in concluding this chapter we have stepped back from the detail of the components of the Profile to consider the wider context of its use. The Profile was conceived and developed as an instrument to be applied to produce data for planning. If that data is to be useful and meaningful, account must be taken of the imperfections of the instrument and of the method of its application, which includes the 'imperfections' - lack of knowledge, inconsistency and emotional involvement - of informants.

10 Applying the data

Identifying the range of needs

The instrument yields a considerable amount of information on needs. There are eight dimensions, each with up to four categories; there are over twelve thousand possible combinations.

The first stage towards using the data is to aggregate it - that is, to add cases together by category in order to get some idea of how many problems there are in each category. This was undertaken for this study by using SPSS-PC. Although in theory it should be possible to do it using an ordinary spreadsheet programme, in practice limitations on the number of cases which can be analysed at a time make it difficult to do so.

The kind of data which are produced by the instrument can be gathered in two different ways. One possibility is for data to be gathered routinely as part of administrative processes, which means that there will be at any time a running record available of needs. The aggregation of needs then becomes a matter of adding or cross-tabulating existing data.

A sample survey, such as those on which our own work is based, presents additional problems. A sample of 10% of a censused population does not necessarily represent one-tenth of the needs of the population. Confidence intervals can be calculated in order to identify the likely range of needs;[1] there is a routine in SPSS-PC, but it does not allow for the use of very small numbers, which is done on the basis of a different set of calculations from that used for larger numbers. The British Medical Journal has issued a computer programme which calculates confidence intervals appropriately.[2] Using that programme, confidence intervals on the rating for behaviour were calculated; they are shown in Table 10.1.

Table 10.1
Estimated numbers with needs related to behaviour on the basis of the sample survey in Tayside

Behaviour: rating of need	Community N	Estimated numbers in the community known to services, 95% ci	Geriatric care N	Estimated numbers in geriatric care, 95% ci
Independent	77	176-260	8	13-57
Long interval	57	124-199	9	16-61
Short interval	74	169-251	18	41-100
Critical interval	88	206-293	58	179-251
Total cases	296		93	

This raises a number of issues for the application of the instrument:

- The calculation of confidence intervals depends on the assumption that the sample will reflect the characteristics of the population. This assumption may be violated, because the population changes rapidly, and between the period of forming the sample frame and making the assessment the cohort will move forward.
- Our sample was large - including, for example, more a third of those in the community - and yet the estimated range is still wide for practical purposes.
- The problems are exacerbated when the base number is small; a difference between 13 and 57 cases (there is an example in this table) could make an enormous difference to the kind of service offered in a locality. Where the number of cases is small, and circumstances are changing rapidly, any planning has to allow for individual circumstances. This implies that it would appropriate to make a budget allocation to cover such contingencies, and to look for subsequent individual assessment, rather than to trying to plan or contract for a service on the basis of these figures.

In the examples which follow, we have referred to figures of those actually sampled rather than the estimated ranges.

Using the data

The kind of information which planners might hope to glean from the instrument will not usually be a simple statement of the numbers of problems. Needs are needs for responses; the instrument provides core information which can be used in order to establish the demand for services.

Two different approaches can be identified; they are likely to be used simultaneously. One addresses the question, 'what is the demand for this service?' The second asks, 'which needs are still unmet after services are allocated, and what should be done about them?' The issues are inter-related; it is fairly clear that the answer to the second depends on the first. In practice the first may also depend on the second: needs which might otherwise be unmet tend to be allocated to existing services (like residential care) because of the absence of alternatives.

Assessing the demand for particular services

The instrument provides more information than is useful for any single service. Although the profile does not make a full assessment of individual need, the number of possible combinations and categories offers planners rather more information than is necessary for most practical purposes. In assessing need for a specific service, therefore, some selection is required.

The process has five main stages:

1. Define the group of people being studied.
2. Exclude people who should have other kinds of service in preference.
3. Select one or two dimensions which are most important to the delivery of the service in question.
4. Compare the level of service required with that offered.
5. Examine the impact of balancing factors and further constraints.

1. Define the group of people being studied The main restriction occurs because the needs of a population have already been met: people in residential care, for example, can be taken not to need home helps, which means that responses from the residential care sector can be excluded from that calculation.

2. Exclude people who should have other kinds of service in preference There are two possible approaches:

- identify a hierarchy of different levels of service, considering the highest levels of service first. People who need the highest level of service will be identified as not requiring lower levels of services - if a person needs full nursing care, then meals on wheels is a poor substitute.
- Identify constraints which would prevent the service being delivered. For example, behaviour, while not a significant element in the determination of needs for housework or the provision of meals, can play a large part in certain cases in deciding whether support at home is appropriate.

It is probably easier to identify service requirements through successive constraints than through the hierarchical approach, but there are arguments for both.

3. Select one or two dimensions which are most important to the delivery of the service in question This is a matter of judgment; we might suggest, for example, that the major factors in the provision of residential care should be behaviour and solitude, while others might take the view that the central issues are carer involvement and problems. Other relevant observations become 'balancing factors' and are dealt with at a later stage.

Some suggested categories for classifying the demand for services are outlined in table 10.2. These are only 'suggested'; the purpose of the instrument is not to prescribe specific options, but to facilitate decision-making.

This process yields a cross-tabulation with a range of dimensions: a 4 x 4 table has sixteen cells. It is possible to incorporate a third dimension - three dimensions with four sub-categories yield 64 combinations - but this is likely to be rather more than necessary.

Table 10.2
Illustrative factors for assessing the demand for services

Service	Dimensions	Balancing factors
Home helps	Domestic tasks	Carer involvement Carer problems
District nurses	Personal care	Carer involvement
Occupational therapy	Personal care	Domestic tasks
Meals	Domestic tasks; solitude	Carer involvement
Residential care	Personal care; behaviour; mobility	Carer involvement Carer problems Solitude
Nursing care	Personal care; mobility; behaviour	
Day care	Solitude; carer problems	
Transport	Mobility; solitude	Material need

4. *Compare the level of service required with that offered* This will indicate whether there is a shortfall or surplus in the level of service.

5. *Examine the impact of balancing factors and further constraints* Although the need for domestic support is the main criterion for referral for home helps, carer problems and solitude might be taken to be influential factors. By excluding those cases in which carers are on hand, a second table can be generated yielding a residual figure - people who need a home help and do not have informal support. In theory, there is no limit to the number of factors which might be considered. In practice, it is rare that a series of balancing factors make much difference.

Priorities It is not our purpose either to propose priorities or to devise an allocations scheme for services. Planners who wish to identify priorities, however, particularly where there are shortages in provision, can do so in the operation of stages (4) and (5). Where (4) indicates a shortage of services, it may be thought desirable to identify a priority group within the totals yielded by (3) by eliminating some people from the calculation - for example, people with a wider range of carers, people with higher material resources, or people with independent mobility.

Example: the demand for home helps

Using the data from the survey material from Tayside makes it possible to produce some illustrative results. The surveys we undertook were not designed to produce a random sample, which means that the figures are not a precise statement of needs, but that is not particularly important for the purposes of a demonstration.

The demand for home helps might be calculated as follows:

1.	*Number of persons assessed while living in the community*	306 (of 917)
2.	*Persons living in the community with problems requiring residential care* (This was calculated for our purposes by saying that a person requires residential care who has critical interval problems in any two of physical, self-care or behaviour.)	47
	Persons remaining in the community	242
	Missing values	17
3.	*Needs for domiciliary care*	
	Independent	22
	Long interval	80
	Short interval	194
	Missing values	10
4.	*Receipt of home help services*	
	Those independent and receiving no home help	16
	Those independent and receiving a home help	6
	Those not fully independent receiving no home help	68
	Those receiving no home help support when short interval help is needed	55

Those receiving long-interval support when short-interval support is needed	45
Those receiving short-interval (daily) support	45
Those receiving short-interval support when long-interval support is needed	14
Those refusing home helps	20
Missing values	5

This shows some shortfall in provision, with some mismatch between needs and the level of services.

5. *Impact of balancing factors*

The effect of considering carer involvement is greatly to mitigate the apparent shortfall in service, though there is some inconsistency in the way support seems to be distributed. Table 10.3 shows the distribution of carer involvement in more detail.

Table 10.3
Carer involvement and the need for domestic support

Need for domestic support	Home help provision			
	None	*Long interval*	*Short interval*	*Refused*
	No carers, or infrequent care			
Independent	2	1	0	1
Long interval	2	12	5	1
Short interval	6	4	9	1
	Long interval support from carers			
Independent	6	4	0	1
Long interval	6	16	5	2
Short interval	4	8	11	1
	Short interval support from carers			
Independent	1	1	0	0
Long interval	5	6	3	1
Short interval	42	31	8	12

The summary figures are:

Those independent and receiving a home help	9
Those not fully independent receiving no care from home help or carer	8 (plus 2 refusals)
Those receiving long-interval support when short-interval support is needed	27
Those receiving short-interval (daily) support	140
Missing values	24

Carer problems Carer problems have (perhaps surprisingly) little effect on these figures. 27 carers had reported both practical and emotional problems, and 5 of these were cases which on other criteria would require residential care. 17 of the remaining 22 had short-interval needs for domestic care. 6 of the 22 were receiving short-interval support, 7 were receiving long interval support, 6 were receiving no support and 3 had refused a home help.

The impact of the need for residential care It is worth reviewing, at this stage, the implications of the decision not to consider the needs of those requiring residential care as part of the demand for home helps. 25 out of 46 for whom data was available were receiving some service, 16 at long intervals and 7 at short intervals; 21 were not, and 2 had refused. This means that some service would become available if these people were allocated residential placements; conversely, if they are not, then there are some outstanding needs which also require to be filled.

Comment

Although the figures are imprecise, they do provide a very clear indication of the direction which policy would need to take in order to meet needs more effectively. The main problem is evidently that people need more frequent domiciliary support than they are in fact receiving. The method makes it possible both to identify the issue and to examine the effects of alternative arrangements.

The method is subject to some important limitations:

- The results are clearly conditional on the assumptions which are made about services.
- There is no way of knowing what proportion of people might refuse services which currently they are not being offered. It follows that even if the perceived shortfall is accurately stated, the effective demand for services cannot be deduced immediately from the figure.
- The instrument does not identify all the needs or demands for

particular services. 'Dementia' refers only to one set of conditions. Most of the services which are available to people with dementia are available for many more needs and conditions besides; one cannot calculate from this instrument the total need for home helps, or for other services like occupational therapy or community psychiatric nursing in a particular area.

- Missing values reduce the sample size through a process of attrition; the more stages which are undertaken in the analysis, the greater the attrition will be. The initial sample covered a third of the people in the community; the figures at stage 5 of the process refer to 218 cases, which when the 47 taken as requiring residential care are included accounts for 86.6% of the sample figure. There is no reason to suppose that missing values necessarily distort the pattern of results, but clearly the effect of moving towards balancing factors is greatly to reduce the number of usable cases.

Determining unmet needs

The next stage is to find out what needs are still unmet after all services have been provided. This can be calculated in two ways. One is to add together services for a group of people - e.g. all those in residential care, or all those in community - and needs for the whole population, and then to take the difference. This is adequate to get a global figure, but in the circumstances of community care it misses an important issue - whether the services are getting to the people they should. This is highly problematic, because it requires a series of judgments to be made about what is the right kind and level of service for each person.

The procedure which has to be followed requires the calculation of residuals after each service has been received. The stages required, for those in community care, are as follows:

1. *Identify people who should not be in community care*, by applying the criteria for residential care.
2. For each category of the profile in turn, *identify which formal services might be considered to meet those needs*, and exclude those cases where such services are available.

   Relevant support for particular categories might include some of the responses in table 10.4.
3. *Identify further whether informal carers can be considered to meet the needs*, not including those cases where carers are not coping, and exclude those cases for which this is true. This applies particularly to personal care, personal care at night, domestic support, behaviour

and behaviour at night. (This stage is optional, because whereas some authorities would consider the services of an informal carer a ground for non-allocation, others would not.)

The remaining figure is the figure for unmet need in that category. The question of whether any one individual has needs which are unmet is fairly complex. For the purposes of planning, the process is rather simpler, and the figures are not difficult to follow. In Tayside, 82 out of 115 people with mobility problems in the community had unmet needs: 37 of these were long interval, 25 short interval and 20 critical interval. 84 out of 155 people with problems in personal care had unmet needs; 40 of these were long interval, 23 short interval and 21 critical interval.

Table 10.4
Illustrative responses to categories of need

Mobility	Occupational Therapy Day Hospital
Personal care	Occupational Therapy Day Hospital District Nurse
Personal care at night	Night sitter
Domestic tasks	Home help Occupational Therapist Day Hospital
Behaviour	Carer involvement
Behaviour at night	Carer involvement Night sitter
Solitude	Day sitters Day centres Lunch clubs
Needs of carers	District Nurse, *and* Respite care *or* Day centres *or* Day hospital

Residential care

For those in residential care, the issues tend to be different. There are usually people in residential care whose circumstances do not warrant the kinds of support which are being offered; if the same criteria were used as those applied above to people in the community, then 279 out of 494 subjects would probably not have been considered to require residential care. However, this assumes a considerable level of support in the community, and discharge is a problematic decision, especially if services in the community are under-developed (as they were in Tayside during this study).

The basic procedure is to identify those who are sufficiently independent not to require residential support. This might be assessed as follows:

1. identify those whose behaviour patterns suggest that they do not require critical interval (or, alternatively, short interval) intervention;
2. identify within this group capacities for personal care and mobility;
3. determine a level of dependency at which residential care is inappropriate (e.g. no more than long interval dependency on any criterion, or short interval dependency on any one factor).

On this basis, of 494 people sampled in residential and hospital care in Tayside there were 29 who were fully independent, and 79 who had no more than long interval dependency, which would make independence possible with very limited support. 54 more had short interval dependency in respect of one factor of personal care or mobility, mainly personal care. If the standard used is less than short-interval need for behaviour, rather than critical interval, the figures are reduced to 25 who are fully independent, 65 with no more than long interval dependency and 29 with short-interval dependency in respect of either mobility or personal care.

Identifying the needs of people in residential care for additional support also requires judgments to be made. Residential and nursing care can be taken to meet most basic needs, including mobility, personal care, domestic care, behaviour and solitude; there is no direct reason to consider the needs of informal carers. At the same time, there are strong arguments for supplementing residential non-nursing services with appropriate health care facilities, particularly from day hospitals and occupational therapists, where these can offer a means of improving the abilities of residents. Of 198 people sampled in non-nursing residential care, in the previous 28 days 5 people were attending day hospital, 9 had seen an occupational therapist, 7 had seen a Community Psychiatric Nurse and 3 had been to day centre.

Responses to unmet needs

Some categories which point to unmet needs might suggest individuated service, while others point to more general gaps in services. From this basic information, it is possible to test out the implications of different service decisions - including both the expansion of existing services, and the development of innovative options - on the total.

The effect of different permutations of services on unmet needs can be modelled incrementally, by trial and error; in principle, it can also be optimised mathematically through linear programming. There are, however, some limitations to precise optimisation. The first is intrinsic to the process of optimisation: there may be more than one optimum. Second, there are normative problems in attaching appropriate weights to costings relative to a range of services which is supposed to be selected for choice, sensitivity, and the achievement of valued but intangible results (like normalisation). And third, there are problems of implementing solutions: there may be no practical way of achieving optima in practice (for example, one cannot realistically abolish residential care altogether, even if an analysis was to suggest it). 'Second best solutions' might be inferior to other possible sub-optima. Rosenhead argues against mathematical optimisation on the basis of uncertain and imprecise data, particularly where there are multiple objectives.[3] Decisions about method need to be made by planners in the context of particular questions to be asked in a specific set of circumstances.

There is also an important practical reservation to make about the accuracy of simulated effects on the residual. The fact that services are supplied with the intention that they should reach people with dementia does not mean that they will ever actually do so. The results of the exercises outlined above suggest that there is a marked shortfall in provision for people who have problems with personal care; but once provision is made in practice, the claims of people with dementia will be balanced by those allocating the services against the claims of others with different but no less pressing conditions. There will often, then, be some 'leakage', and it may be necessary to make some allowance for this.

Mismatches in needs and services

The instrument can also be used to identify whether there are mismatches between the needs of the population and the services which are being provided. The first procedure, identifying the demand for a service, yields a figure of how much of a service is required. The second procedure indicates the extent of unmet need, by category. Where there is unmet need and a surplus of provision, or where unmet need is greater than the shortage, there is some mismatch of needs and services. Where the level of unmet need is lower than the apparent demand for a service, it is probably because some other services, or informal carers, are substituting for the service which is being examined.

11 Ethical issues

Ethical approval was sought for this project at the outset from the local heath service research ethics committee, and the project was approved. Because it involved no invasive procedures, and because it effectively duplicated many activities routinely undertaken in the planning and organisation of services, the ethical dimensions of the study initially seemed marginal. In practice, however, a number of ethical issues arose, and it is important for those wishing to undertake similar activity to review them here.

Ethical issues relating to planning studies

Research which is devoted to the development of planning procedures is unusual in health care, and at the outset there was little guidance available on ethical practice which was directly applicable to a project of this kind. The Mental Health Commission, in its guidance on Consent to Treatment, also considers a number of aspects of the ethics of research. They distinguish 'therapeutic' research - research from which the patient stands to benefit from an intervention - from 'non-therapeutic' research; they suggest that non-therapeutic research requires much more rigorous safeguards, and indeed that in many cases of people with mental impairments that such research should not be undertaken at all, because they are unable to give full informed consent. This, Murphy suggests, would 'outlaw' most research with people with dementia at a stroke.[1] But, she argues, the test is too restrictive:

> any research that leads to a better understanding of the patient's condition is part of the doctor's obligation to his patients and hence part of the therapeutic role.[2]

Planning to meet people's needs is not strictly speaking 'therapeutic'. But it is done in the service of therapeutic activity, and the primary justification for the project is that the procedures which are being developed can be used to improve the extent to which services are available to meet needs. (The process of identifying needs may also yield a secondary benefit, by alerting professionals to some individual problems.)

Planning studies share with epidemiological studies a common characteristic: that they examine the features of a population.

- The focus of such studies is social rather than individual. The concern is to identify issues relating to populations rather than to benefit individuals.
- The persons who are studied are not necessarily those who will benefit.
- Data are collected and processed which refer to the characteristics of the population.

Studies of a population are in consequence subject to two important ethical objections:

- Information is necessarily collected about persons who cannot benefit from the research.
- The process requires the use of personal information over which each individual has rights.

If data collection is subject to general rules which govern research activity, then individuals should have the right to withdraw from the research, and their consent should be sought. This is the substance of a draft directive from the European Commission on data protection; there has been concern that the effect of such procedures may be to make much medical research impossible.[3] The idea that people have rights over the content of research derives from a particular view of the research relationship. The idea of consent, in particular, has been drawn from legal practice in the US. Kennedy argues that the basis of this doctrine, which he refers to as 'transatlantic', is a concern with the autonomy of subjects.[4] The ethical objections describe ethical considerations rather than the *sine qua non* for research (or indeed for medical treatment), and while there is a presumption in their favour they have to be balanced against other considerations.

Planning studies can be justified in a number of ways (for example, it can be argued that social issues should be considered paramount over individual ones), but many are not compatible with the liberal and individualistic principles associated with Western medicine. The most important justifications tend, in consequence, to be utilitarian ones. This can be represented to mean that:

a. an act is justified if the benefits to some exceed the costs to others (the principle behind cost-benefit analysis); or
b. an act is justified if it makes some people better off without making

any others worse off (a principle generally accepted in welfare economics[5]); or

c. an act if justified if some people benefit and the costs to the losers are minimal.

The problem with (a) is that the costs to others may be unacceptably high. Principle (b) is unexceptionable on individualistic grounds (though it is sometimes disputed where it leads to undesirable distributional consequences). It is closely compatible with an axiom which has been described as fundamental to medical ethics - *primum non nocere*, that the first duty of the doctor is to do no harm.[6] However, it is difficult to envisage circumstances in which no costs are imposed on anyone as a result of a study. The effect is that principle (c) obtains most generally, with some trade-off being made between the potential costs to losers against the perceived benefits of the study. There is however a clear ethical duty to minimise such costs where they arise.

The implications of this argument are that a study must seek to identify the marginal costs and benefits to the people who are the subject of the research. The process of collecting material for planning purposes generally involves very low costs to individual subjects.

- Data can be collected and applied routinely from the normal patterns of operational activity.
- Data can be collected without any intrusion into the private circumstances of individuals.
- Individuals often stand to benefit personally from the process, which serves to monitor and safeguard current practice as well as to provide information for future activity.

By contrast, collecting material for research, or the purposes of piloting a planning process, is subject to a range of problems. There are marginal costs to the people whose information is being recorded, in terms of time taken and the intrusiveness of inquiries. There may be marginal benefits - our researchers felt, as professional social workers, that the interviews with carers often proved to have a beneficial or supportive effect - but these are uncertain, and they cannot be relied on. The primary justification must be that the marginal cost is sufficiently small to be outweighed by the benefits. To achieve this we sought:

- to obtain information as far as possible from people who would already be in possession of the data;
- to obtain the information in a manner which would minimise disturbance or cost to the subjects of the research; and
- to process and use the information in a manner which implied no costs to the subjects of the research.

Ethical issues relating to people with dementia

The deterioration of intellectual faculties implies that people with dementia become progressively less able to retain new information, and so to absorb it. Dementia reduces a person's will and directed activity, and the ability of a person with dementia to behave autonomously. The deterioration of emotional faculties becomes evident in behavioural disturbance, emotional lability, passivity and inappropriate reactions. None of this implies that people with dementia should be considered prima facie incapable of making decisions. The argument for treating people with dementia with respect depends partly on the belief that everyone has to be treated with a degree of basic respect,[7] and partly on the practical argument: people with dementia may be aware, and even if they are not there are problems of distinguishing those who are not from those who are. In the case of care for elderly people, we are only beginning to be aware of some of the same kinds of abuses and problems which affect other groups who are stigmatised or considered 'non-persons'. Rights and respect are fundamental to the protection of people from abuse. Marshall proposes the following principles of action:

1. People with dementia have the same human value as anyone else irrespective of their degree of disability or dependence.
2. People with dementia have the same varied human needs as anyone else.
3. People with dementia have the same rights as other citizens.
4. Every person with dementia is an individual.
5. People with dementia have the right to forms of support which do not exploit family and friends.[8]

Informed consent

It is generally required in most kinds of research for the informed consent of the subjects to be sought. Informed consent includes explanation of four main factors:

- what the research is about
- who is financing the research
- the purposes of the research
- how the research will be disseminated

as well as awareness of the subjects' right to refuse to participate.[9]

There are often difficulties in doing this in relation to planning or epidemiological research. A refusal to participate, for example, would render the process of a census impossible. The Council for International Organizations of Medical Sciences *International Guidelines for Ethical Review of Epidemiological Studies*[10] state that:

> Individuals or their public representatives should normally be told that their data might be used in epidemiological studies, and what means of protecting confidentiality are provided.

The British Medical Association has commented that:

> Although the general rule is that the subject's consent must be obtained for any disclosure of personal health information, in the case of some kinds of health research this may sometimes not be reasonably practicable (e.g. in epidemiological research in which studies do not necessarily involve any contact with the individuals concerned).[11]

There is then a presumption that informed consent will be obtained, but it is defeasible. There are two principal circumstances in which the general rule might not obtain. The first, noted by the BMA, is that there are circumstances in which obtaining such consent is not reasonably practicable and no contact with the subject is required. For example, it would not normally be considered unethical to conduct a traffic survey to see what proportion of drivers were wearing seat belts. If Kennedy is right to argue that the root of the doctrine of informed consent rests in a concern with the autonomy of the subjects,[12] the reason why this kind of practice is acceptable is that, provided it is subject to appropriate safeguards, it presents no threat to autonomy within the law. If we had been concerned with a different kind of subject group, such as smokers or athletes, the combination of not requiring personal contact with practical difficulties might have been conclusive; but the particular vulnerability of people with dementia to abusive procedures argues for a more stringent test.

The second exception to the presumption that informed consent should be obtained is the case in which the research may prove distressing to subjects. The *International Guidelines* recognise that in general, 'prospective subjects ... might feel needlessly anxious about why they were subjects of study.' Feeling 'needlessly anxious' is probably not a sufficient objection to a full explanation of the procedures, though it is worth emphasising that seeking consent from people who are not being directly studied can in normal circumstances puzzle and alarm them. Of greater concern is the proviso made by the BMA that 'no damage or distress will be caused to the subject of the information.' The particular circumstances of dementia suggest a potential for creating real distress. In particular:

- the effect of referring to dementia, or asking questions about memory loss or behaviour, can be to alert people with dementia or their carers to the fact that the issue is in question;

- the impact of asking personal questions about behaviour or continence can be intrusive and distressing;
- the effect of investigating relationships and behaviour can be to alter those relationships;
- people suffering from dementia are likely to experience some distress when being questioned in terms they feel they cannot answer; and
- the process of referral could damage the relationships of the person with dementia or carer with the referring professional.

By contrast, the potential personal benefit to those who offer co-operation is low. Identifying memory or behavioural problems offers no direct benefit to people with dementia or carers; it may even be perceived, with some reason, as threatening, because the terminology is associated with a loss of autonomy. In addition, the population with dementia is unusually fluid. The work we have done on the flow of people with dementia, supra, suggests that many if not most will be in different circumstances within two years of a study. This emphasises the general point which applies in other epidemiological studies, that those who are being studied are not likely to be those who benefit.

The literature did not offer clear guidance about circumstances of this kind. Smith and Nichols[13] review the issues in obtaining the consent to research in relation to dementia, but they are concerned only with therapeutic and non-therapeutic research which involves the direct participation of the person with dementia, and they do not consider the possibility of research which requires information about the person but does not require their participation. We looked, then, to discussions of the ethics of research in other related fields.

In sociological research, unlike most medical research, it is often possible to approach research problems through the understanding of intermediaries. The British Sociological Association's Statement of Ethical Practice is particularly geared to circumstances, like that of this project, where the focus of concern falls on social rather than individual factors, and takes particular note of the circumstances of vulnerable respondents. They recommend that sociologists should strive to :

1. ensure that the physical, social and psychological well-being of research participants is not adversely affected by research;
2. protect the rights of those they study (including their interests, sensitivities and privacy) ...
16. anticipate any harmful effects on the participants as a consequence of the research process
17. minimise the disturbance on the participants that results from the research process
18. be particularly careful where research participants are vulnerable

because of their age, social status or powerlessness

19. avoid intruding on the personal space of the ill, very young or elderly and frail (and where suitable use informants or intermediaries to provide the data).[14]

There is still a general recommendation within these guidelines to obtain consent, and subjects should have the opportunity not to participate in research. At the same time, in the specific case of those who are vulnerable, it may be appropriate to obtain information through intermediaries. There is however a potential conflict here; the process of obtaining informed consent can itself involve a considerable intrusion. There are besides particular practical difficulties in obtaining informed consent from people with dementia: their loss of comprehension, and problems with factual recall, can make it difficult to be sure that real informed consent has been obtained.

Our main ethical concerns in compiling the data were:

- to minimise the distress to respondents
- to minimise the costs to people with dementia, and
- to minimise the intrusiveness of the procedure.

The tests which are applicable to the censuses and survey work undertaken for this project are slightly different. In relation to the censuses:

- there was no need to refer to individual subjects
- there was no evident risk to the autonomy of subjects in making the enquiry
- there were practical difficulties in obtaining the consent of subjects, and
- the process of obtaining consent would have threatened the integrity of the census.

In the case of the assessment of needs:

- there was considerable risk of intrusion in relation to the personal circumstances of subjects
- there was the potential to generate distress by asking personal questions, or by communicating a specific interest in dementia; and
- there was also no need to refer to individual subjects.

We did not use the term 'dementia' in the course of negotiating access or obtaining information. Interviews were conducted solely by our researchers, both trained and experienced social workers. In cases where people with dementia were present during an interview, the interviewers discussed issues with them according to circumstances; in other cases, we sought to minimise contact with people suffering from dementia themselves. The main exception to this approach, which is noted in chapter 9, was the attempt to test the possibility of a small number of interviews with people who had dementia. This was tackled sensitively, and discontinued when it proved ineffective for the purposes of the research.

In taking the decision to minimise contact, we also decided not to seek the consent of people with dementia. While recognising the force of the argument for obtaining consent, we faced a moral dilemma; the protection of people with dementia argued for minimal disruption and contact, and consent could not be obtained without more than that minimal disruption and some risk. We discussed the issue of consent at great length within our own group, and ultimately had to balance considerations about the rights of people with dementia against a powerful set of objections. It was unnecessary to involve people with dementia in most of our inquiries, and there was no evident risk to their autonomy if we did not do so, but there was a potential to cause distress if we did. On that basis, the majority of our group felt it was inappropriate to seek consent.

Ethical issues relating to carers

The position of carers throws up many of the same kind of issues. Carers have a distinct moral status which requires recognition. However, even a spouse cannot undertake many legal relations on behalf of the other partner. In the US, the principle that a proxy can consent to research has been advocated, notably by the National Commission for the Protection of Human Subjects.[15] Dworkin, reviewing the literature, notes that this has been controversial; proxies do not necessarily act in the subject's interests.[16] In the UK, the principle of the proxy has never been accepted. Twigg comments:

> despite the established practice of consultation, relatives in fact have no legal status in medical decision-making and this extends to spouses. ... Issues arise, however, where the patient is mentally incapable, for example by reason of severe mental illness, learning disability or organic brain damage through senile dementia or a stroke. Often in such cases the individual is cared for by a relative, who perforce has to make decisions for them on a day-to-day basis. The legal basis for such decision-making is, however, far from certain. ... Where an adult is incapable of giving consent, there is no clear alternative source. ... The consent of a relative 'is of no effect since there is no power vested in a relative to consent to the treatment of another'.[17] Machinery does exist whereby decisions can be made in regard to property, but this does not extend to decisions concerning the person.[18]

The practice of seeking consent from relatives can be regarded as a safeguard -

Jonsen argues that someone has to make an assessment about the risk of harm[19] - but it is not sufficient for ethical purposes. The practice of seeking consent from relatives is widespread, but it rests on no firm ethical or legal base.

We also wished, though, to obtain information from informal carers, both as subjects in their own right and as informants about the people they were caring for. Informal carers were consulted only in circumstances where they were to be primary informants. This applied only to the survey of the needs of people in the community, approximately one in six of those on whom we had obtained some information. The considerations which apply to people with dementia applied no less to carers: we had

- to minimise the distress to respondents
- to minimise the costs, and
- to minimise the intrusiveness of the procedure.

We needed the consent of the carer in so far as we were asking the carer to co-operate by giving us information, and in doing so observed other ethical guidelines - including explanation of the purpose of the study, guaranteeing anonymity and confidentiality, and permitting respondents to refuse participation. We did not use the term 'dementia', because we were concerned with symptomatology rather than formal diagnosis, and the consent we sought was in terms of those symptoms. In cases where carers were not aware of an existing diagnosis of dementia, the effect of communicating it would have been

- to have breached confidentiality of information held about the subject
- to have disturbed relationships with professionals, and
- to have faced the informal carer with information which might change the relationship of that person to the subject.

The procedures for contacting respondents are described in chapter 9. The guiding principle was to avoid causing any upset or distress to the carer: if the professional advised against contact this advice was taken. In two circumstances procedures we had intended to investigate more fully were dropped at early stages when we felt they caused distress to carers. These were the initial attempt to conduct interviews over the telephone, and the request to carers to keep a detailed diary of events.

Ethical issues relating to professionals

Professionals were our main source of information, in two respects. First, information from professionals was the basis on which the census of people with dementia was made. Second, professionals often responded as the principal carers of people with dementia, particularly but not solely for people in residential care and hospital.

The initial identification of sufferers proved to be the most controversial aspect of the research, and a number of professionals, including psychiatrists, psychiatric nurses, doctors working in medicine for the elderly, and voluntary organisations, expressed concern about it. There is an argument that information gained in the context of a professional relationship (e.g. doctor-patient) is confidential to that relationship and should not be passed to a third party unconnected with the direct care of the patient or client. This is not generally accepted or practised: the Department of Health's recent draft guidelines clearly consider records-based research of this type to be legitimate. The Department of Health argues that this process is justified in terms of the benefits to the NHS and the public health.

> Patients implicitly authorise that their records, including health information obtained from other sources, will be used by the NHS and Department of Health for wider NHS purposes which are essential to the delivery of high quality health care to themselves and the population as a whole. The wider NHS purposes include ...
> - clinical research ...
> - the management and planning of services ...
> - (and) statistical purposes in support of both clinical and management functions.[20]

This is a fairly robust statement, which tends to suggest that there is no fundamental ethical difficulty in undertaking research of this kind. The information required needed some unique identifier in order to identify multiple returns; furthermore, the primary purpose of the census is to create a sample frame and anonymous data would be unsuitable for this. In most cases (but not in all) the effect of contact and discussion was to allay the concerns expressed. It is important to recognise, however, that these concerns are consonant not only with traditional concerns about confidentiality but also with the principles currently being applied in data protection - that information which is obtained for one purpose cannot be released for another without the consent of the person to whom it applies. The argument relates, then, to a general principle, and it is not specific to the field of dementia. The issue is one which will need to be resolved by everyone working in this field if epidemiological work is to continue.

There is a second potential issue, relating to the identification of needs in the sample. There is an ethical problem (equivalent to that faced by informal carers) of whether it is legitimate and consistent with professional relationships to reveal the specific details of a case without the consent of the person. We were aware, having made a finely balanced decision about this, that objections might be raised, and the arguments are reviewed above. The issue, perhaps surprisingly, did not arise; those who were likely to raise it in the course of the survey had done so more generally in relation to the census.

Safeguards

The BMA's suggestions for safeguards for the use and disclosure of personal health information have been incorporated in a draft Bill.[21] The Bill is concerned primarily with disclosure of data from medical records and is directly relevant to the census stage and to completion of survey assessment forms by staff in longstay care establishments. The BMA argues that disclosure is acceptable:

> where the disclosure is approved by an appropriate ethics committee, for the purpose of health service research, and there are safeguards to ensure that no damage or distress will be caused to the subject of the information and that the results of the research are not made available in a form which identifies the subject.

Further safeguards suggested in the draft Bill include:

- Consent to use the data should be obtained from the relevant qualified health professional.
- No approach should be made to the subject about whom data has been disclosed without the consent of the responsible qualified health professional.
- Data should not be disclosed to anyone outside the research team.
- Data should be destroyed when no longer required for the approved research.

The approach of the Tayside surveys followed both the spirit and the letter of the guidance offered in this draft Bill.

The benefits of the research

Much of the argument which has been presented here is based partly on a importantly pessimistic premise: that the direct benefits to the subjects of the research will be limited. Viewed in individualistic terms, this is probably true, and it is important to be able to justify the research in such terms if individuals are to be protected adequately. But it is also worth qualifying this proposition by some consideration of the social value of research for service planning. Social values cannot adequately be arrived at by examination of the consequences for each individual. The issue is not so much that some people will gain at the expense of others, but that some people bear costs in order for others to benefit. There is in society a 'norm of reciprocity'.[22] Reciprocity implies not that people give in order to receive, but that social exchange relationships can be seen in terms of a pattern of 'generalized reciprocity' or 'social solidarity' in which the returns made are indirect.[23] Pensions are paid for by a current generation of workers in the expectation that their children will pay in turn for their pensions. One of the justifications for this kind of research - a justification which is often referred to informally in the process of seeking consent - is that it will benefit people later, as people now are helped by the contributions of people who co-operated with research in the past. The costs experienced by people with dementia, carers and professionals cannot be disregarded; if there were no benefits from a project like this one, even the most minimal costs would imply that intervention was not justifiable. The perception of relationships of social solidarity can help to some extent to mitigate the costs which some people undergo for the benefit of others.

Appendix

The potential permissions which could be sought, and the procedures followed in Tayside, are shown in the table below.

Table 11.1
Consents sought

	Census			**Survey**		
	Community	*Residen-tial*	*Hospital*	*Community*	*Residen-tial*	*Hospital*
Person with dementia	No contact	No contact	No contact	No contact	No contact	No contact
Carer/ relative	No contact	No contact	No contact	Consent obtained subsequent to professional agreement	No contact	No contact
Professional	Consent obtained	Consent obtained	Consent obtained	Consent obtained	Consent obtained	Consent obtained

12 Conclusion

The purpose of the project described in this book was to develop and pilot a new approach to collecting data for planning purposes. In chapter 3, we outlined a number of criteria by which the profile would have ultimately to be judged.

Validity Validity concerns the question of whether the profile measures the things we think it does. The main justifications for considering that it does are theoretical rather than empirical: if we are wrong to identify needs in terms of functional dependency, clearly the data which are produced would not represent needs but something else. The other main issue to note is that we did not focus very strongly on the diagnosis of dementia, choosing instead to identify people with dementia-like conditions. We felt for planning purposes that a more precise distinction is untenable in terms either of planning or of service responses. If particular conditions inducing dementia (like, say cerebrovascular disease) were to prove susceptible to a cure, it would become important to distinguish such conditions from others prior to any other decisions about the allocation of resources.

Even if the theoretical basis is sound, there is the possibility that there is something about the method which leads to measurements being made of different issues from those which are intended. There are a number of cautionary notes to make.

- The recognition of problems is not truly independent of the service received. It is possible that services inculcate a degree of dependency -if people do not cook for themselves, for example, they may lose such abilities as they have. One important difficulty which emerged in the fieldwork was the inability of staff in residential homes to identify the capacities of people with dementia in tasks they were not normally asked to do.

- The kinds of response which people give are sometimes guided by what they consider the consequences to be. Carers often minimise difficulties because they are fearful of the consequences, for example the removal of a loved spouse to residential care. Conversely, people who really want a service may feel impelled to stress their problems.
- People's perceptions of their circumstances may be unclear. If carers find the process of keeping a diary depressing, it may be because they have not previously faced the issues related to the behaviour of the person with dementia. The answers which people give can be affected by their desire to show themselves or others in a particular light.
- There are often conflicts of interest between the sufferer and the carer; there may be financial considerations attached to the reactions of residential care.

These are important issues, which would have to be faced in any attempt to measure the needs of old people. The tests for reliability can show that we are getting consistent results, but of course that may mean that we are getting consistently distorted results. The main defence of the procedure we have adopted is that it will still produce useful indicators; figures should never be taken to represent reality so exactly that they can be relied on as the sole basis for decisions.

Reliability The issue of reliability has been extensively reviewed in chapter 9. This shows the instruments used to be generally reliable (in the sense of producing consistent results) under certain conditions. In principle, the importance of reliability is much less than that of validity: consistent information is not meaningful if people reliably report figures which are useless anyway. The main purpose of the extensive checks we performed was to see whether or not the instrument held up under different conditions.

Two important issues emerged here. The first is that the circumstances of people with dementia change rapidly, and the information which is given is sometimes uncertain on that basis. Second, respondents do not always know sufficient information about the person they are answering for. There are important differences in the judgments made by professionals and informal carers, and the decision to obtain information from one source rather than another can have a large effect on the data obtained.

Ease of application and use Unlike some other assessment instruments, we have finished with a fairly short, and we believe a fairly simple, process. The costings were difficult to establish with confidence in our field trials, because so much time was spent in examining alternatives and retesting, but in Forth Valley, where the instrument has subsequently been applied, the full cost (including the costing of staff time) amounted to £10,000, of which aproximately one-quarter was attributable to the census and three-quarters to the assessment.

Fitness for purpose We have established that the instrument can be used as the basis for allocative decisions. We cannot specify exactly how it will be used, because that depends on the range of services which is provided, the perceived role of those services and the priorities of planners. Many other issues play a part in such decisions - most obviously, finance. Decision making is a complex activity, which is rarely reducible to a simple technical process. The most we can argue, then, is that the information is in a form which can contribute to decision making.

Adaptability The profile is adaptable in two main ways. The first is built into the design of the instrument. Different factors can be used in different permutations for different purposes. There is a limit to how sophisticated this analysis can be, because at each stage when the data are processed there is some loss of usable information; but there is a very large number of possible permutations which are available for analysis of material in outline.

The second way in which the instrument might be modified is externally. There is the scope to add in further dimensions; if, for example, stimulation and education were identified as implying functional needs, or if one felt there should be a category for the emotional distress of people with dementia, the method by which such dimensions might be incorporated is clear. Equally, we believe that the basic method we have used should be adaptable to a range of other types of need besides dementia.

Robustness We knew, when we started this project, that scales of any type have an unhappy history. Whatever the cautions which the designers make, whatever is said about the process of application, people in the field ignore it. We have said that the instrument should not be used for individual assessments. We have no way of making sure that it never is; all we can say is that if it is used for individual assessments, those assessments will probably not be very good.

We tried to make the scale as 'bomb-proof' as we could. In particular, we tested the scale out to see how far it could be applied by different people in different settings. We developed, as a result, two main ways of compiling a profile: the identification of categorisations by specially trained staff, and the use of more specific questions with informal carers. Attempts to use existing professional staff with minimal briefing were less successful - not in the main because of problems of reliability, but because they tended to leave holes in the information. The best protection appeared to be to approach informal carers, which called for the use of closed, simply worded questions rather than the more open, qualitative assessment sought from professionals. It is worth noting even so that the results were most reliable when delivered by trained professionals conducting interviews on the basis of those broadly-framed questions.

The Tayside Profile makes it possible for the data necessary for service planning to be collected efficiently and effectively, in ways which are adaptable to local circumstances. It produces the data in a form which can be applied for different purposes, and it does it at relatively low cost. The best justification for an instrument of this sort is that it works; this one does.

Notes

Notes to chapter 2

1. World Health Organisation, 1980, International Classification of Impairment, Disabilities and Handicaps, Geneva: WHO.
2. The phrase is from Townsend P, 1979, Poverty in the United Kingdom, Harmondsworth: Penguin.
3. Roth M, 1981, The diagnosis of dementia in late and middle life, in Mortimer J, Schuman L, The epidemiology of dementia, New York: Oxford University Press, p 24.
4. Kitwood T, Bredin K, 1992, Towards a theory of dementia care, Ageing and Society 12(3) pp 269-287.
5. Gilleard C J, 1984, Living with dementia, Croom Helm.
6. Zarit S, Todd P, Zarit J, 1986, Subjective burden of husbands and wives as caregivers, Gerontologist 26(3) pp 260-266.
7. Sanford J, 1978, Tolerance of debility, in Carver V, Liddiard P (eds.), An ageing population, Hodder and Stoughton.
8. Jones K, 1985, After hospital, University of York Department of Social Policy and Social Work.
9. Argyle N, Jestice S, Brook C, 1985, Psychogeriatric patients: their supporters' problems, Age and Ageing 14 pp 355-360.
10. Gilleard C J, 1984, Problems posed for supporting relatives of geriatric and psychogeriatric day patients, Acta Psychiatrica Scandanavica, 70 pp 198-208.
11. Gilleard C J, Boyd W, Watt G, 1982, Problems in caring for the elderly mentally infirm at home, Archives of Gerontology and Geriatrics, 1, p 157.
12. Levin E, Sinclair I, Gorbach P, 1989, Families, services and confusion in old age, Aldershot: Avebury.

13. Feinberg J, 1973, Social philosophy, Prentice Hall, Englewood Cliffs NJ.
14. See O'Connor D, Pollitt P, Brook C, Reiss B, 1989, A community survey of mental and physical infirmity in nonagenarians, Age and Ageing 18 pp 411-414.
15. Pollitt P, Anderson I, O'Connor D, 1991, For better or for worse: the experience of caring for an elderly dementing spouse, Ageing and society, 11, pp 443-469.
16. Pollitt et al., 1991, p 468.
17. Social Services Inspectorate /Social Work Services Group, 1991. Care management and assessment, HMSO.
18. Jones K, 1985.
19. Blumenthal M, Journal of Clinical Experimental Gerontology 1979; cited Norman A, 1982, Mental illness in old age, Centre for Policy on Ageing.
20. E.g. Nevitt A A, 1977, Demand and need, in Heisler H (ed.), Foundations of social administration, London: Macmillan; Williams A, 1974, "Need" as a demand concept, in Culyer A J (ed.), Economic problems and social goals, Oxford: Martin Robertson.
21. Spicker P, 1993, Needs as claims, Social Policy and Administration 27(1) pp 7-17.
22. Bradshaw J, 1972, A taxonomy of social need, in G McLachlan (ed.) Problems and progress in medical care, 7th series, Oxford University Press.
23. The literature on the problems created for carers is substantial; reviews of the literature include Fadden G, Bebbington P, Kuipers L, 1987, The burden of care, British Journal of Psychiatry, 150: 285-292; Parker G, 1990, With due care and attention, FPSC; and Twigg J, Atkin K, 1994, Carers perceived, Buckingham: Open University Press.
24. Bayley M, 1973. Mental handicap and community care, RKP, London.
25. Spicker P, 1989. Social Housing and the Social Services, Longmans.
26. Gilhooly M, 1987. Senile dementia and the family, in J Orford (ed.) Coping with disorder in the family, Beckenham: Croom Helm, p 158.
27. See Campbell A, McCosh L, Reinken J, Allan B, 1983. Dementia in old age and the need for services, Age and Ageing 12 pp 11-16.
28. Gilhooly, 1987, pp 159-160. See also O'Connor D, Pollitt P, Brook C, Reiss B, Roth M, 1991, Does early intervention reduce the number of elderly people with dementia admitted to institutions for long term care?, British Medical Journal 302 pp 871-75.

29. Faludi A, 1973. Planning theory, Pergamon; Pendreigh D, Planning a systematic approach, in Kinnaird J et al., The provision of care for the elderly.
30. Falk N and Lee J, Planning the social services, 1978; Faludi, 1973.
31. Lindblom C, The science of muddling through, in Faludi A (ed.) 1973, A reader in planning theory, Pergamon.
32. Griffiths R, 1988, Community care: agenda for action, HMSO.
33. Etzioni A, 1973, Mixed scanning: a third approach to decision making, in Faludi A (ed.), A reader in planning theory, Oxford: Pergamon.
34. Williams A, Anderson R, 1978, Efficiency in the social services, Martin Robertson.
35. Spicker P, 1987. Concepts of need in housing allocation, Policy and politics 15(1) 17-27.
36. Norman A, 1982. Mental illness in old age, Centre for Policy on Ageing.
37. Melzer D, Hopkins S, Pencheon D, Brayne C, Williams R, 1992, Epidemiologically based needs assessment report 5: Dementia, NHS Management Executive.
38. Melzer et al., 1992.
39. See Jones D, Vetter N, 1985, Formal and informal support received by carers of elderly dependants, British Medical Journal 291 7.9.85 643-645; and O'Connor D, Pollitt P, Brook C, Reiss B, 1989, The distribution of services to demented elderly people living in the community, International Journal of Geriatric Psychiatry, 4 pp 339-344. By contrast, Levin et al., 1989, do seem to find a general increase in some services as dementia is more serious, though this is not closely related to need.
40. McCafferty P, 1994, Living independently, Department of the Environment, ch 4. The assessment of dependency is based on the scale used by Bond and Carstairs, discussed at greater length in chapter 4 of this book.
41. Wakeford report, 1984, Sheltered housing for older people, Age Concern, p 38.
42. Thornton P, Mountain G, A positive response, Joseph Rowntree Foundation 1992, pp 24-25.
43. Challis D, 1989, Elderly dementia sufferers in the community, in Morton J (ed.) Enabling elderly people to live in the community, Age Concern Institute of Gerontology, London.

Notes to chapter 3

1. Kane R A, Kane R L, 1981. Assessing the elderly, Lexington, Mass.: Lexington Books.
2. Carley M, 1981. Social measurement and social indicators, Allen and Unwin.
3. Henderson A, Huppert F, 1984, The problem of mild dementia, Psychological Medicine, 14 pp 5-11; Mowry B, Burvill P, 1988, A study of mild dementia in the community using a wide range of diagnostic criteria, British Journal of Psychiatry 153 pp 328-34.
4. Henderson A, 1986. The epidemiology of Alzheimer's disease, British Medical Bulletin, 42(1) pp 3-10.
5. Copeland J et al., 1992, Alzheimer's disease, other dementias, depression and pseudodementia: prevalence, incidence and three-year outcome in Liverpool, British Journal of Psychiatry 161 pp 230-239.
6. Bickel H, Cooper B, 1994, Incidence and relative risk of dementia in an urban elderly population, Psychological Medicine 24 179-192.
7. Boothby H, Blizard R, Livingston G, Mann A, The Gospel Oak Study state III: the incidence of dementia, Psychological Medicine 24 89-95.
8. Copeland et al., 1992.
9. Jorm A, Henderson A, Kay D, Jacomb P, 1991, Mortality in relation to dementia, depression and social integration in an elderly community sample, International Journal of Geriatric Psychiatry 6(1) pp 5-11.
10. Gordon D S, Gillies B, McWilliam N, Spicker P, 1993, A local census of dementia sufferers, Scottish Medical Journal, 38(6) pp 186-187.
11. Goda D, 1985, Pathways into and between services for the elderly in Scotland, Unpublished report to Scottish Home and Health Department.
12. Knopman D, Kitto J, Deinard S, Heiring J, 1988, Longitudinal study of death and institutionalisation in patients with primary degenerative disorder, Journal of the American Geriatrics Society 36(2) pp 108-112.
13. Kay D, 1991, The epideomiology of dementia, Reviews in Clinical Gerontology 1 pp 55-66.
14. Ineichen B, 1987, Measuring the rising tide, British Journal of Psychiatry, 150 pp 193-200.

Notes to chapter 4

1. Wilkin D, 1987, Conceptual problems in dependency research, Social Science and Medicine, 24(10) pp 867-73.

2. Pattie A, Gilleard C, 1979, Clifton Assessment Procedures for the Elderly.
3. See Wilkin D, Thompson C, 1989. Users' guide to dependency measures for elderly people, University of Sheffield Joint Unit for Social Services Research.
4. McGrother C, Jagger C, Clarke M, Castleden C, 1990, Handicaps associated with incontinence: implications for management, Journal of Epidemiology and Community Health 44 pp 246-48; Teri L, Larson E, Reifler B, 1988, Behavioral disturbance in dementia of the Alzheimer's type, Journal of the American Geriatrics Society 36, 1-6.
5. Pattie and Gilleard, 1979, p 7.
6. Thompson Q, 1973, Assessing the need for residential care in the elderly, GLC Intelligence Bulletin 24.
7. Bond J, Carstairs V, 1982, Services for the Elderly, Scottish Home & Health Department, Edinburgh.
8. Finklestein V, 1993, From curing or caring to defining disabled people, in Walmsley J, Reynolds J, Shakespeare R, Woolfe R (eds.) Health, welfare and practice, London: Sage, p 142.
9. Isaacs B, Neville Y, 1975, The Measurement of Need in Old People. Scottish Home & Health Department, Edinburgh.
10. Bond and Carstairs, 1982.
11. Askham J and Thompson C, 1990, Dementia and Home Care. ACIOG, London; Gilhooly M, 1984, The social dimensions of senile dementia, pp 88-135 in Hanley I and Hodge J (eds.) Psychological Approaches to the Care of the Elderly, London: Croom Helm; Morris R, Morris L, Britton P, 1988, Factors affecting the emotional wellbeing of the caregivers of dementia sufferers, British Journal of Psychiatry, 153: 147-156.
12. Black J, 1985, Care Network Project: First Findings: The Networks of Care of Elderly Demented People in the Community - Instrumental Care. Working Paper 37, Department of Social Theory and Institutions, UCNW, Bangor.
13. Marshall M, 1993, New trends and dilemmas in working with people with dementia and their carers, in Chapman A, Marshall M (eds.) Dementia: new skills for social workers, London: Jessica Kingsley, p 8.
14. Argyle N, Jestice S, Brook C, 1985, Psychogeriatric patients: their supporters' problems, Age and Ageing, 14: 355-360; Askham J, Thompson C, 1990, Dementia and Home Care, London: ACIOG Research Paper 4; Gilhooly M, 1984, The impact of care-giving on care-givers: factors associated with the psychological well-being of people supporting a dementing relative in the community, British

Journal of Medical Psychology 57 pp 35-44; Gilleard C, 1984, Problems posed for supporting relatives of geriatric and psychogeriatric day patients, Acta Psychiatrica Scandinavica, 70 pp 198-208; Gilleard C, Belford H, Gilleard E, Whittick JE, Gledhill K, 1984, Emotional distress amongst the supporters of the elderly mentally infirm, British Journal of Psychiatry, 145 pp 172-177; Gilleard, Boyd, Watt, 1982; Morris et al., 1988; O'Connor D, Pollitt P, Roth M et al., 1990, Problems reported by relatives in a community study of dementia, British Journal of Psychiatry 156: 835-841; Rabins D, Mace N, Lucas M, 1982, The impact of dementia on the family, Journal of American Medical Association 248 pp 333-335; Zarit S, Reever K, Bach-Peterson J, 1980, Relatives of the impaired elderly: correlates of feelings of burden, Gerontologist 20 pp 649-655.

15. Greene J, Smith R, Gardiner M, Timbury G, 1982, Measuring behavioural disturbance of elderly demented patients in the community and its effects on relatives: a factor analytic study, Age and Ageing, 11 pp 121-26.
16. Isaacs and Neville, 1975, p 1.8
17. Anderson R, 1987, The unremitting burden on carers, British Medical Journal, 294 p 73; Jackson J, Anderson D, Cambridge P (1986) The experiences and needs of carers of the elderly mentally infirm, Social Services Research, 15 pp 95-127; Jones D, Vetter N (1984) A survey of those who care for the elderly at home: their problems and their needs, Social Science and Medicine, 19 pp 511-514; Levin E, Sinclair I, Gorbach P, 1989 Families, Services and Confusion in Old Age. Aldershot: Avebury; McCullough D, 1989, The Needs of Carers of Elderly People with Dementia. Strathclyde Regional Council, Glasgow; Parker G, 1990, With Due Care and Attention: A Review of Research on Informal Care, London: Family Policy Studies Centre, London.
18. Poulshock S and Diemling G, 1984, Families caring for elders in residence: issues in the measurement of burden, Journal of Gerontology, 39 pp 230-39; Vitaliano P, Young H, Russo J, 1991 Burden: a review of measures used among caregivers of individuals with dementia, Gerontologist, 31 pp 67-75.
19. Wright F, 1986, Left to Care Alone. Aldershot: Gower.
20. Silliman R, Sternberg J, 1988, Family caregiving: impact of patient functioning and underlying causes of dependency, Gerontologist, 28 pp 377-382.
21. Askham J, Grundy E, Tinker A, 1992, Caring: The importance of third age carers, Dunfermline: Carnegie UK Trust.

22. Wilkin D, Thompson C, 1989, Users' Guide to Dependency Measures for Elderly People, Sheffield: Joint Unit for Social Services Research.
23. Askham J, 1991, The problem of generalizing about community care of dementia sufferers, Journal of Aging Studies 5 pp 137-146.

Notes to chapter 5

1. Jorm A, Korten A, Henderson A, 1987, The prevalence of dementia: a quantitative integration of the literature, Acta Psychiatrica Scandinavica, 1987 pp 465-479.
2. Hofman A, Rocca W, Brayne C, Breteler M et al., 1991, The prevalence of dementia in Europe, International Journal of Epidemiology 20(3) pp 736-748.
3. See C J Gilleard, 1984, Living with dementia, Beckenham: Croom Helm.
4. O'Connor D, Pollitt P, Hyde J, Fellows J et al., 1989, The prevalence of dementia as measured by the Cambridge Mental Disorders of the Elderly Examination, Acta Psychiatrica Scandinavica 79 pp 190-98.
5. See e.g. Levin E, Sinclair I, Gorbach P, 1989, Families, Services and Confusion in Old Age, Avebury, Aldershot; National Consumer Council, 1991, Consulting Consumers in the NHS: A Guideline Study: Services for Elderly People with Dementia Living at Home, NCC, London.

Notes to chapter 6

1. Annual Report, Registrar General Scotland; Scottish Health Statistics (annual); Community Care Bulletin 1991 (CMC2/1993), Social Work Services Group, January 1993; Community Care Plan, Social Work Department, Tayside Regional Council, September 1993 (update); Census 1991 Report for Tayside Region and Report for Scotland.
2. Data was obtained from: Annual Report, Registrar General Scotland; Scottish Health Statistics (annual); Community Care Bulletin 1991 (CMC2/1993), Social Work Services Group, January 1993; Community Care Plan, Social Work Department, Tayside Regional Council, September 1993 (update); Census 1991 Report for Tayside Region and Report for Scotland.
3. Kay D, 1991, The epidemiology of dementia: a review of recent work, Reviews in Clinical Gerontology 1 pp 55-66; Miller N, Cohen G, 1981, Clinical aspects of Alzheimer's Disease and senile dementia:

synopsis and future perspectives in assessment, treatment and service delivery, in Miller N and Cohen G (eds.) Clinical Aspects of Alzheimer's Disease and Senile Dementia, Raven Press, New York.
4. Black S, Blessed G, Edwardson J, Kay D (1990) Prevalence rates of dementia in an ageing population: are low rates due to the use of insensitive instruments? Age and Ageing, 19 pp 84-90; Copeland J, 1990, Suitable instruments for detecting dementia in community samples, Age and Ageing, 19 pp 81-83; Kay, 1991.
5. Brayne C, Ames D, 1988, The epidemiology of mental illness in old age, in Gearing B, Johnson M, Heller T (eds.) Mental Health Problems in Old Age, Wiley, Chichester; Henderson A, Huppert F, 1984, The problem of mild dementia, Psychological Medicine, 14 pp 5-11; Kay, 1991; Mowry B, Burvill P, 1988, A study of mild dementia in the community using a wide range of diagnostic criteria, British Journal of Psychiatry 153 pp 328-34.
6. Clarke M, Jagger C, Anderson J, Battcock T et al., 1991, The prevalence of dementia in a total population: a comparison of two screening instruments, Age and Ageing, 20 pp 396-403; Henderson and Huppert, 1984.
7. Blessed G, 1989, Definition and classification of the dementias: the point of view of a clinician, in Wertheimer J, Baumann P, Gaillard M, Schwed P (eds.) Innovative Trends in Psychogeriatrics, Basel: Karger; Brayne C, Calloway P, 1990, The association of education and socio-economic status with the Mini-mental State Examination and the clinical diagnosis of dementia in elderly people, Age and Ageing, 19 pp 91-96; Herbst K, Humphrey C, 1980, Hearing impairment and mental state in the elderly living at home, British Medical Journal, 281 pp 903-5; O'Connor D, Pollitt P, Hyde J, Fellowes J et al., 1991, The progression of mild idiopathic dementia in a community population, Journal of American Geriatrics Society, 39 pp 246-51; O'Connor D, Pollitt P, Treasure F, 1991, The influence of education and social class on the diagnosis of dementia in a community population, Psychological Medicine 21 pp 219-24.
8. Bond J, 1987, Psychiatric illness in later life: a study of prevalence in a Scottish population, International Journal of Geriatric Psychiatry 2 pp 39-57; Henderson A, 1986, The epidemiology of Alzheimer's Disease, British Medical Journal, 42, 3-10; Kay D, 1991, The epidemiology of dementia: a review of recent work, Reviews in Clinical Gerontology 1 pp 55-66.
9. Jorm A, Korten A, Henderson A, 1987, The prevalence of dementia: a quantitative integration of the literature, Acta Psychiatrica Scandinavica, 76 pp 465-79.

10. Hofman A, Rocca W, Brayne C, Breteler M et al., 1991, The prevalence of dementia in Europe: a collaborative study of 1980-1990 findings, International Journal of Epidemiology 20 pp 736-48.
11. Brayne C, Ames D, 1988, The epidemiology of mental illness in old age, in Gearing B, Johnson M, Heller T (eds.) Mental Health Problems in Old Age, Chichester: Wiley.
12. Bond J, Carstairs V, 1982, Services for the Elderly, Scottish Home and Health Department, Edinburgh; cf Brooks P, 1992, Planning services for dementia, Health Bulletin, 50 pp 206-215.
13. Carr J, 1992, Tayside Dementia Services Planning Survey, Stirling: Dementia Services Development Centre.
14. Blessed G, 1988, Long stay beds for the elderly severely mentally ill, Bulletin of the Royal College of Psychiatrists 12 pp 250-52.
15. Martyn C, Pippard E, 1988, Usefulness of mortality data in determining the geography and time trends of dementia, Journal of Epidemiology and Community Health 42 pp 134-37.

Notes to chapter 7

1. Barer B, Johnson C, 1990 A critique of the caregiving literature, Gerontologist, 30 pp 26-29; Schulz R, Visintainer P, Williamson G, 1990, Psychiatric and physical morbidity effects of caregiving, Journal of Gerontology, 45 pp 181-91.
2. E.g. Gilleard C J, Gilleard E, Gledhill K, Whittick J, 1984), Caring for the elderly mentally infirm at home: a survey of supporters, Journal of Epidemiology and Community Health, 38 pp 319-25; Lewis J, Meredith B, 1988, Daughters Who Care: Daughters Caring for Mothers at Home, Routledge, London.
3. Wright F, 1986, Left to Care Alone. Aldershot: Gower.
4. Charlesworth A, Wilkin D, Durie A, 1984, Carers and Services: A comparison of men and women caring for dependent elderly people, Manchester: Equal Opportunities Commission.
5. Dura J, Kiecolt-Glaser J, 1990, Sample bias in caregiving research, Journal of Gerontology 45 pp 200-4.
6. Barer and Johnson, 1990; Goodman C, 1986, Research on the informal carer: a selected literature review, Journal of Advanced Nursing, 11 pp 705-712.
7. Gallagher D et al., 1989, Prevalence of depression in family caregivers, Gerontologist, 29 pp 449-56; O'Connor D, Pollitt P, Brook C, Reiss B, 1989, The validity of informant histories in a community

study of dementia, International Journal of Geriatric Psychiatry, 4 pp 203-8; Schulz et al. 1990.

8. Badger F, Cameron E, Evers H, 1990, Waiting to be served, Health Service Journal 11 Jan pp 54-5; Slipping through the net, Health Service Journal 18 Jan pp 86-7.
9. McCullough D, 1980, The Needs of Carers of Elderly People with Dementia, Glasgow: Strathclyde Regional Council.
10. Levin E, Sinclair I, Gorbach P, 1983, The Supporters of Confused Elderly Persons at Home: Volume 3: Appendices, London: National Institute of Social Work; Levin E, Sinclair I, Gorbach P, 1989, Families, Services and Confusion in Old Age, Avebury: Aldershot. The two reports give different figures.
11. Levin E, Sinclair I, Gorbach P, 1989, Families, Services and Confusion in Old Age, Avebury: Aldershot.
12. Levin et al. 1989.
13. Courtesy of Professor Mary Marshall and John Carr, Dementia Services Development Centre, University of Stirling.
14. Pollitt P, O'Connor D, Anderson I, 1989, Mild dementia: perceptions and problems. Ageing and Society 9 pp 261-75; Pollitt P, Anderson I, O'Connor D, 1991, For better or for worse: the experience of caring for an elderly dementing spouse, Ageing and Society 11 pp 443-469.
15. Folstein M, Folstein S, McHugh P, 1975, Mini Mental State: a practical method for grading the cognitive state of patients for the clinician, Psychiatric Research 12 pp 189-198.
16. Greene J et al., 1982, Measuring behavioural disturbance of elderly demented patients in the community and its effects on relatives: a factor analytic study, Age and Ageing 11 pp 121-126.
17. Jorm A, Jacomb P, 1989, The Information Questionnaire on Cognitive Decline in the Elderly (IQCODE): socio-demographic correlates, reliability, validity and some norms, Psychological Medicine 19 pp 1015-1022.
18. Estimates were pro rata estimates from cases solely identified by responding GPs and geriatric continuing care wards. These were made by place of residence and 'non-dementing' rates by place of residence were then applied to the estimated number.
19. Livingston G, Hawkins A, Graham N et al., 1990, The Gospel Oak study: prevalence rates of dementia, depression and activity limitation among elderly residents in Inner London, Psychological Medicine 20 pp 137-146.
20. O'Connor D, Pollitt P, Hyde J, Fellows J et al., 1989, The prevalence of dementia as measured by the Cambridge Mental Disorders of the Elderly Examination, Acta Psychiatrica Scandinavica 79 pp 190-98.

21. Levin et al., 1989, p 10.
22. Levin et al., 1989, p 191.
23. Iliffe S, Booroff A, Gallivan S et al., 1990, Screening for cognitive impairment in the elderly using the mini-mental state examination, British Journal of General Practice, 40 pp 277-9; Ineichen B, 1989, Senile Dementia: Policy and Services, Chapman and Hall, London; O'Connor D, Pollitt P, Hyde J, et al., 1988, Do general practitioners miss dementia in elderly patients?, British Medical Journal 297 pp 1107-10; Philp I, Young J, 1988, An audit of a primary care team's knowledge of the existence of symptomatic demented elderly, Health Bulletin 46 pp 93-7; Smith A, Robertson R, Bishop M, 1984, An assessment of the elderly patients in a new town general practice, Health Bulletin, 42 pp 234-51.
24. Jacques A, 1988, Understanding Dementia, Edinburgh: Churchill Livingston, p 72.
25. Kay D, Beamish P, Roth M, 1964, Old age mental disorders in Newcastle upon Tyne, British Journal of Psychiatry 110 pp 146-58.
26. Gordon D, Spicker P, 1996, Demography, needs and planning: the challenge of a changing population, in Hunter S (ed.) Research highlights - Dementia, London: Jessica Kingsley (forthcoming).
27. Tayside Regional Council Social Work Department, 1988, Towards Better Care: An issue paper reviewing the Social Work Department's residential care services for elderly people, Dundee:TRC.

Notes to chapter 8

1. Beech J, Harding L (eds.), 1990, Assessment of the Elderly, Windsor: NFER-Nelson; Jorm A, Jacomb P, 1989 The Informant Questionnaire on Cognitive Decline in the Elderly (IQCODE): socio-demographic correlates, reliability, validity and some norms, Psychological Medicine, 19 pp 1015-22; Jorm A, Korten A, 1988, Assessment of cognitive decline in the elderly by informant interview, British Journal of Psychiatry, 152 pp 209-13; Jorm A, Scott R, Jacomb P, 1989, Assessment of cognitive decline in dementia by informant questionnaire, International Journal of Geriatric Psychiatry, 4 pp 35-39; O'Connor D, Pollitt P, Brook C, Reiss B, 1989, The validity of informant histories in a community study of dementia, International Journal of Geriatric Psychiatry 4 pp 203-208; Roth M, Tym E, Mountjoy C, Huppert F et al., 1986, CAMDEX: A standardised instrument for the diagnosis of mental disorder in the elderly with special reference to the early detection of dementia, British Journal of

Psychiatry 149 pp 698-709.
2. Askham J, 1995, Making sense of dementia: carers' perceptions, Ageing and Society 15 pp 103-114.
3. Levin et al., 1989.
4. Levin et al., 1989, p 29.
5. Martin J, Meltzer H, Elliot D, 1988, The Prevalence of Disability among Adults, London: OPCS. Melzer D, Hopkins S, Pencheon D, Brayne C, Williams R, 1992, Dementia, Epidemiologically Based Needs Assessment Report 5 (provisional version), London: NHS Management Executive, cite unpublished work by Opit using this scale to make estimates regarding dementia.
6. Levin E, Sinclair I, Gorbach P, 1983, The Supporters of Confused Elderly Persons at Home: Volume 3: Appendices, London: National Institute of Social Work.
7. Askham J, Thompson C, 1990, Dementia and Home Care. London: Age Concern Institute of Gerontology; Bergmann K, Foster EM, Justice A, Matthews V, 1978), Management of the demented elderly patient in the community, British Journal of Psychiatry, 132 pp 441-49; Gilleard C, Gilleard E, Gledhill K, Whittick J, 1984, Caring for the elderly mentally infirm at home: a survey of supporters, Journal of Epidemiology and Community Health 38 pp 319-25; Goda D, 1985, Pathways into and between services for the elderly in Scotland, Unpublished Final Report to Scottish Home and Health Department; Lindsey J, Murphy E, 1989, Dementia, depression and subsequent institutionalisation - the effect of home support, International Journal of Geriatric Psychiatry 4 pp 3-9.
8. Levin E, Sinclair I, Gorbach P, 1989, Families, Services and Confusion in Old Age, Aldershot: Avebury.
9. Marshall M, 1994, A home for life?: profiling of People with Dementia for Long-stay care, Edinburgh: Scottish Action on Dementia.

Notes to chapter 9

1. Clarke M, Jagger C, Anderson J, Battcock T, et al., 1991, The prevalence of dementia in a total population: a comparison of two screening instruments, Age and Ageing 20 pp 396-403; Reisberg B, Ferris S, Steinberg G et al., 1989, Longitudinal study of dementia patients and aged controls: an approach to methodologic issues, in Lawton M, Herzog A (eds.) Special Research Methods for Gerontology, Amityville NY: Baywood Publishing.

2. Joint Centre for Survey Methods, 1991, Telephone Surveys, JCSM Newsletter, 11(3) p 3.
3. Herzog A, Kulka R, 1989, Telephone and main surveys with older populations: a methodological overview, in Lawton M, Herzog A (eds.) op cit.
4. Cotrell V, Schulz R, 1993, The perspective of the patient with Alzheimer's Disease: a neglected dimension of research, The Gerontologist 33 pp 205-11.
5. Gillies B, 1995, The Subjective Experience of Dementia. Department of Social Work, University of Dundee.
6. Gamsu C, 1983, A corrected version of the calculation of weighted Kappa and its associated statistics. mimeo.
7. Calculated after Gamsu C,. op cit, using weights recommended by Cicchetti D and Sparrow S, 1981, Developing criteria for establishing interrater reliability of specific items: applications to assessment of adaptive behaviour, American Journal of Mental Deficiency 86 pp 127-137.
8. Cicchetti and Sparrow 1981.
9. Cicchetti and Sparrow 1981.
10. Bond J, Carstairs V, 1982, Services for the Elderly, Edinburgh: Scottish Home and Health Department, pp 124-125.
11. Ong K, Nolan M, 1994, Assessment and community care: are the reforms working? Generations Review, 4 pp 2-4.
12. Urquhart J (Information and Statistics Division, Scottish Health Service), personal communication, March 1995.
13. Brace S, Buckley G, Hunter S, Samuel E, 1991, Process and Preference: Assessment of Older People for Institutional Care. Final Report to Chief Scientist Office, Scottish Office Home and Health Department, University of Edinburgh.

Notes to chapter 10

1. The methods are described in M J Gardner, D G Altman, 1989, Statistics with confidence: confidence intervals and statistical guidelines, London: British Medical Journal.
2. S Gardner, P Winter, M J Gardner, 1991, Confidence interval analysis, London: BMJ Publishing.
3. J Rosenhead, 1978, Operational research in health services planning, European Journal of Operational Research, 2 pp 75-85.

Notes to chapter 11

1. Murphy E, 1986, Psychiatric implications, in Hirsch S, Harris J (eds.) Consent and the incompetent patient, London: Gaskell/Royal College of Psychiatrists, p 71.
2. Murphy, 1986, p 71.
3. See Wald N, Law M, Meade T, Miller G, Alberman E, Dickinson J, 1994, Use of personal medical records for research purposes, British Medical Journal 309 26th November pp 1422-1424.
4. Kennedy I, 1988, Treat me right, Oxford: Clarendon Press.
5. Little I, 1957, A critique of welfare economics, Oxford: Oxford University Press.
6. Jonsen A, 1977, Do no harm: axiom of medical ethics, in Spicker S F, Englehardt H (eds.) Philosophical medical ethics, Dordrecht, Netherlands: Reidel.
7. Downie R, Telfer E, 1980. Caring and curing: a philosophy of medicine and social work (London, Methuen); Spicker P, 1990, Mental handicap and citizenship, Journal of Applied Philosophy 7(2) pp 139-151.
8. Marshall M, 1990. Working with dementia: guidelines for professionals, Birmingham: Venture Press, pp 10-12.
9. British Sociological Association, Statement of Ethical Practice, 1991.
10. CIOMS. International Guidelines for Ethical Review of Epidemiological Studies. Geneva: CIOMS, 1991.
11. British Medical Association, 1994, Commentary on *Disclosure and Use of Personal Health Information Bill*, London: BMA.
12. Kennedy, 1988.
13. Smith A, Nichols D. Dementia: Consent to Research. Edinburgh: Scottish Action on Dementia, 1992.
14. British Sociological Association, 1991, Statement of Ethical Practice: reproduced in Harvey L, McDonald M, 1993, Doing Sociology, Macmillan, p 4.
15. National Commission for the Protection of Human Subjects in Biomedical and Behavioural Research, 1978, Research involving those institutionalised as mentally infirm, cited Dworkin R, 1992, Researching persons with mental illness, London: Sage, p 78.
16. Dworkin, 1992.
17. Citation of Kennedy, 1988.
18. Twigg, 1994, p 284.
19. Jonsen, 1977, p 35.
20. Department of Health, 1994, Draft guidance for the NHS on confidentiality, use and disclosure of personal health information,

London: Department of Health.
21. *Disclosure and Use of Personal Health Information Bill*, HL Bill 37, London: HMSO, 1996.
22. Gouldner A, 1960, The norm of reciprocity, American Sociological Review 25(2) pp 161-177.
23. Mauss M, 1925, The Gift, London: Cohen and West; Ekeh P, 1974, Social Exchange theory, London: Heinemann; Heath A, 1976, Rational choice and social exchange, Cambridge: Cambridge University Press.

Appendix

The forms and guidance notes developed for use in the research programme

This appendix contains the material included in four forms, with guidance notes where applicable. They are

- the form for people in community care
- the form for people in hospital
- the form for people in residential care, and
- the questionnaire for carers.

For the purposes of presenting the information here, the size of the original print has been reduced; columns are presented consecutively, rather than side-by-side; and space left for notes and written information has been minimised. In the original format, the community care form covered four sides of paper (a folded A3 paper, presented as an A4 folder); the hospital form covered two sides of A4 paper, with material on the second side being for short-term patients only; the residential care form covered one side of A4 paper; and the questionnaire for carers covered eight sides, with an additional page provided for comments.

Community care

Guidance for filling the form
(see also Guidance Booklet)

Page 1 contains information for filing purposes. The space at the bottom right is for a file name.

Pages 2-4 ask for an assessment of needs. There is space for notes on the left of the page. On the right, you may be asked to choose a code. Numbers or letters should be *circled* (or written in when appropriate).

Some examples have been given as indications of the kind of things being looked for in each category, but they are not the only kinds of factor which might be relevant.

Additional problems can be written in the Notes section. The space for Notes on this page can be used for any general information which might be relevant or useful, including details about any medical condition which might affect the sufferer's abilities.

Definitions

Ratings are based on the level of help/monitoring required, regardless of whether the dependency is brought about by physical or mental incapacity, or both. If there are problems which occur in more than one category, the highest rating should be chosen. All ratings are based on the current situation at the time of rating.

Carer:
Used as shorthand for the informal care network, which may be a lone carer or several carers co-operating.

Help:
This refers to personal assistance/supervision from anyone which is needed for an activity to be performed adequately or behaviour monitored. Use of aids does not count as help. Drugs are treated as aids - if a problem is controlled by drugs, then it is not rated as a current problem.

Notes:

<table>
<tr><td colspan="2">Ref:</td><td colspan="2">CONFIDENTIAL</td></tr>
<tr><td colspan="4">Surname</td></tr>
<tr><td colspan="4">First names</td></tr>
<tr><td>Date of Birth</td><td colspan="2">Age</td><td>Sex</td></tr>
<tr><td colspan="4">Address</td></tr>
<tr><td colspan="4"></td></tr>
<tr><td colspan="4">Tel:</td></tr>
<tr><td colspan="4">Type of accommodation:</td></tr>
<tr><td></td><td colspan="2">Sheltered housing</td><td>1</td></tr>
<tr><td></td><td colspan="2">Other formal supported housing</td><td>2</td></tr>
<tr><td></td><td colspan="2">All other housing</td><td>3</td></tr>
<tr><td colspan="4">Referred to study by:</td></tr>
<tr><td colspan="4">Name of respondent:</td></tr>
<tr><td colspan="3">Address and tel. if different from above:
....
....
....</td></tr>
<tr><td colspan="3">Date of assessment:</td></tr>
</table>

<table>
<tr><td rowspan="4">Physical mobility
[Mobility means the physical ability to move around, rise from a chair and so forth. There is a question later about problems of wandering or getting lost. People are likely to need help from anyone at long intervals if they have difficulties walking outside; they are likely to need help at critical intervals if they have problems walking indoors.]
Notes</td><td>INDEPENDENT
No help needed</td><td>0</td></tr>
<tr><td>INFREQUENT
Help needed less than once a week</td><td>1</td></tr>
<tr><td>LONG INTERVAL
Help needed once a day or less.</td><td>2</td></tr>
<tr><td>CRITICAL INTERVAL
Help needed more than once a day.</td><td>3</td></tr>
<tr><td rowspan="6">Self care and continence
[This section refers to activities such as dressing, washing, bathing or assistance with the toilet. The main question concerns how frequently people need help from anyone with such activities. Problems with bathing or dressing tend to be long interval (once a day) or short interval (more than once a day). Where a person is incontinent, the question to be asked is whether it is possible to help on a plannable basis (short interval), or if the incontinence is unpredictable or very frequent (critical interval).]
Notes</td><td>INDEPENDENT
No help needed.</td><td>0</td></tr>
<tr><td>INFREQUENT
Help needed less than once a week</td><td>1</td></tr>
<tr><td>LONG INTERVAL
Help needed once a day or less.</td><td>2</td></tr>
<tr><td>SHORT INTERVAL
Help needed more than once a day, at regular times.</td><td>3</td></tr>
<tr><td>CRITICAL INTERVAL
Help needed more than once a day, either at unpredictable times, or very frequently.</td><td>4</td></tr>
<tr><td>NIGHT
Help with personal care needed at night</td><td>N</td></tr>
</table>

Need	Level	Score
Need for domestic support [This refers to ordinary housework such as shopping, washing and ironing, cleaning and dusting, cooking, or making a hot drink. Help from anyone with shopping is usually done at long intervals (once a day or less); help from anyone with housework or laundry tends to be long interval (once a day or less) but can be short interval (more than once a day); help from anyone with meals is usually short interval (more than once a day). *The question you should ask is not whether the person with dementia actually does these things, but whether help from anyone is needed, and if so how frequently.*] *Notes*	**INDEPENDENT** No help needed.	0
	INFREQUENT Help needed less than once a week	1
	LONG INTERVAL Help needed once a day or less.	2
	SHORT INTERVAL Help needed more than once a day.	3
Behaviour [This section asks whether a person has a need for help from anyone either because of certain actions, or because that person fails to act. There are very many kinds of behaviour which might cause a problem: examples might include apathetic behaviour - e.g. being inactive, not eating disturbed or disruptive behaviour - e.g. day-night reversal, shouting, inappropriate sexual behaviour or endangering behaviour - wandering, careless use of cigarettes. Ratings should be based on *how often* a carer would be required to deal with problems of behaviour, including having to "keep an eye on" the sufferer.] Please make a brief note of the problems here. *Notes*	**INDEPENDENT** Help or monitoring is not needed.	0
	INFREQUENT Help needed less than once a week	1
	LONG INTERVAL Help or monitoring is needed once a day or less.	2
	SHORT INTERVAL Help or monitoring is needed more than once a day, but at regular times.	3
	CRITICAL INTERVAL Help or monitoring is needed more than once a day, either at unpredictable times, or very frequently (more than every two hours).	4
	NIGHT Help is needed during the night.	N

Who is caring? [These questions are about informal carers - family, friends or neighbours who give help without payment. Please do not include paid services such as home help or district nurse.] *Notes*	How many main informal carers are there?	
	Do any of the main informal carers live with the sufferer? Answer Y (yes) or N (no).	
	Relationship of carer(s) to sufferer.	
	Age of carer(s)	
	Gender of carer(s)	
	Do the carer(s) have any other informal support (ie. from other relatives, friends, etc)? Answer Y (yes) or N (no).	
Carer Involvement [This section is concerned with the length of time that the informal carers are actually involved in caring tasks either with, or on behalf of the sufferer.] *Notes*	**NONE** This is to be marked when there is no *informal* carer.	0
	INFREQUENT The time burden or disruption for carer is less than once a week.	1
	LONG INTERVAL Carer involved once a day or less.	2
	SHORT INTERVAL Carer involved more than once a day, on a *plannable* basis.	3
	CRITICAL INTERVAL Carer involved more than once a day, either frequently or on an unpredictable basis.	4
	NIGHT Carer involved at night.	N

Are the carers coping? [This asks about two different kinds of problems. *Practical* problems which are likely to affect caring include the ill health of the carer, threat to employment, competing family commitments, financial difficulties. *Emotional* problems include feelings of distress, poor morale, friction between carers, isolation. This section *refers to the situation of the main informal carer.*] *Notes*	**COPING** Is the main carer coping? Answer Y (Yes) or N (No)	
	PRACTICAL ISSUES Are there practical problems as a result of helping or caring? Answer Y (Yes) or N (No).	
	EMOTIONAL ISSUES Is the carer upset by the situation? Answer Y (Yes) or N (No).	
Social isolation of the sufferer [This section is trying to establish how long the sufferer is *at home* alone during the day. A day will normally be from morning to evening (7 a.m. to 10 p.m.).] *Notes*	**NOT ISOLATED** Usually alone for less than 5 hours in a day.	1
	MODERATE ISOLATION Usually alone for between 5 and 10 hours in a day.	2
	ISOLATED Usually alone for more than 10 hours per day.	3

Material resources of sufferer: **House tenure** *Notes*	Owner-occupier	1
	Rented or other secure tenure.	2
	Other	3
House condition [Amenities include any of: inside wc, hot water, bath/shower, central heating.] *Notes*	No problems.	1
	Lacking amenities or major disrepair.	2
Income *Notes*	Basic state pension/income support.	1
	plus special disability/care benefits.	2
	plus private income (occupational pension, investment income).	3
	plus special benefits *and* private income.	4

Formal services [Please write in *number of days* in past 4 weeks service has been received by sufferer *or* carer on behalf of sufferer. The aim is to find out what kind of support is currently being provided; approximate answers will do. If service has been offered but refused please enter "R".] *Notes*	General Practitioner	
	District Nurse	
	Health visitor	
	Community psychiatric nurse	
	Continence Service	
	Social Worker or Care Manager	
	Occupational therapist	
	Home help or social care officer	
	Meals on wheels	
	Laundry service	
	Night Sitter	
	Day Sitter	
	Day Hospital (name):	
	Day Centre (name):	
	Lunch Club	
	Carer's Group	
	Other, eg. Voluntary Groups (specify)	
Respite care [This asks whether the sufferer has been in respite care - like a residential home, nursing home, hospital for a holiday, in order to give the carer a break.]	Has the sufferer had respite care during the last year? Answer Y (Yes) or N (No).	
	If yes, has this been on a regular basis? Answer Y (Yes) or N (No).	

Guidelines for Needs Assessment Profile (Community Care)

The Profile has been designed for use by local Health and Social Work planners to assess the needs of people with Dementia. It is not intended to provide individual assessments but to provide information on levels of need in the population as a whole.

User Guide

The aim of the profile is to identify the needs of the dementia sufferer in relation to physical mobility, self care and continence, domestic support, behaviour and carer burden, and to indicate at what level help is needed.

The profile is intended to be administered by a range of people eg. social workers, home helps, community nursing staff, day care officers etc., in a variety of settings and is not dependent on the training of staff.

The Profile

Reference: This should be left blank for administrative purposes.

Details of **Names, Date of Birth,** etc., refer to the dementia sufferer who is being assessed.

Type of Accommodation

Sheltered Housing This refers to Local Authority, private or voluntary sheltered housing.
Other formal supported housing This refers to to other combinations of housing, such as housing supported by neighbourhood services; combinations linking residential/community housing; very sheltered housing; cluster housing or alms houses.
All Other Housing This refers to house owner; council tenant; privately rented; owned by someone else (eg. a relative such as son/daughter)

Referred to study. This refers to name of person who provided sufferer's name

Name of respondent This refers to name of person completing form.

Date of assessment This refers to date form is completed.

Areas Measured

Many of the areas measured use the concept of **the interval** (independent, infrequent, long, short, critical), which is the time during which an individual can cope without help or attention. The person who completes the form is being asked to make an assessment of how frequently help is needed.

Examples have been given in the areas of **Physical Mobility, Self care and**

continence, Need for domestic support and **Behaviour**, but there are many possibilities; the answer should be based on how frequently intervention is needed.

Who is caring, Carer involvement, and **Are the the carers coping** refer to main informal carers such as family, friends or neighbours not paid services.

Social isolation of the sufferer refers to how long the sufferer is alone at home during the day.

MATERIAL RESOURCES OF THE SUFFERER

House Tenure

This refers to whether sufferer/spouse owns house; rents it; shares another's house (eg. a relative such as a son or daughter).

House Condition

This refers to lack of facilities in the house which make caring difficult:
- e.g. inside toilet; hot water; bath/shower or central heating,
or
- whether the house requires a lot a major repairs.

Income

This refers to whether, as well as basic pension/income support, the sufferer :
- receives any special benefits eg. Attendance Allowance
and/or
- receives any private income from savings/investments or occupational pension.

Formal Services

This measures the range and frequency of services being received. If, for example, a District Nurse has called twice a week over the past month, the number "8" should be entered. If the G.P. has visited once during the time, enter "1". If the sufferer has attended any Day Centre, Club etc., enter the number of visits and the name of the establishment visited.

Respite Care

This refers to any period of time the sufferer spends away from home, to give the carer a break.

People in hospital

Confidential	Ref:	
Surname:		
First names		
Date of Birth	Age	Sex
Hospital and ward		
Tel:		
Type of ward:		
	Psychiatric	1
	Medicine for the Elderly	2
	Other	3
Name and status of respondent		
Date of assessment		

Guidance for filling the form
(see also Guidance Booklet)
Numbers or letters above should be circled.

If the patient is short-term, or being considered for discharge, complete both sides. As a general guideline, a patient who has has been in hospital for less than two months should be treated as short-term.

If a patient is a long-term resident, fill only the first page.

Notes
Use this space for any general information which might be relevant or useful, including details about any medical condition which might affect the sufferer's abilities.

Physical Mobility	
Independent No help needed	1
Long interval Help needed once a day or less	2
Critical interval Help needed more than once a day	3
Self Care and Continence	
Independent No help needed	1
Long interval Help needed once a day or less	2
Short interval Help needed more than once a day, at regular times	3
Critical interval Help needed more than once a day, unpredictably or very frequently	4
Night Help needed with personal care at night	N
Need for Domestic Support	
Independent No help needed	1
Long interval Help needed once a day or less	2
Short interval Help needed more than once a day	3
Behaviour	
Independent No help needed	1
Long interval Help/monitoring needed once a day or less	2
Short interval Help/monitoring needed more than once a day at regular times	3
Critical interval Help needed more than once a day, unpredictably or very frequently	4
Night Help/monitoring needed at night.	N

Support in the community

(to be answered only for short term patients, or those being considered for discharge.)

Informal care	
How many main informal carers are there?	
Do any of the main informal carers live with the sufferer? Answer Y (yes) or N (no).	
Relationship of carer(s) to sufferer.	
Age of carer(s)	
Gender of carer(s)	
Do the carer(s) have any other informal support (ie. from other relatives, friends, etc)? Answer Y (yes) or N (no).	

Carer involvement	
NONE This is to be marked when there is no informal carer.	0
INFREQUENT The time burden or disruption for carer is less than once a week.	1
LONG INTERVAL Carer involved once a day or less.	2
SHORT INTERVAL Carer involved more than once a day, on a *plannable* basis.	3
CRITICAL INTERVAL More than once a day, either frequently or unpredictably.	4
NIGHT Carer involved at night	N

Can the carers cope?	
COPING Can the main carer cope? Answer Y (Yes) or N (No)	
PRACTICAL ISSUES Does caring pose practical problems? Y (Yes) or N (No).	
EMOTIONAL ISSUES Is the carer upset by the situation? Answer Y (Yes) or N (No).	

Patient's Home Address:

Social Isolation of the sufferer	
NOT ISOLATED Usually alone at home for less than 5 hours in a day.	1
MODERATE ISOLATION Usually alone at home for between 5 and 10 hours in a day.	2
ISOLATED Usually alone at home for more than 10 hours per day .	3
Accommodation	
Independent housing	1
Supported housing (e.g. warden)	2
Residential care	3
No accommodation currently available	4
Material resources of sufferer: Housing tenure	
Owner-occupier	1
Rented or other secure tenure.	2
Other	3
Material resources: House condition	
No problems.	1
Lacking amenities or major disrepair.	2
Material resources: Income	
Basic state pension/income support.	1
plus special disability/care benefits.	2
plus private income (occupational pension, investment income).	3
plus special benefits *and* private income.	4

Guidelines for Needs Assessment Profile

(People in Hospital)

The Profile has been designed for use by local Health and Social Work planners to assess the needs of people with Dementia. It is not intended to provide individual assessments but to provide information on levels of need in the population as a whole.

User Guide

The aim of the profile is to identify the needs of the dementia sufferer in relation to physical mobility, self care and continence, domestic support, and behaviour and to indicate at what level help is needed. If a patient is short-term or likely to be discharged, then carer burden is also assessed.

The form should be completed by a member of the Hospital Staff who is familiar with the dementia sufferer. A separate form should be completed for each sufferer being assessed.

The Profile

Reference: This should be left blank for administrative purposes.

Details of **Name, Date of Birth,** etc., refer to the dementia sufferer who is being assessed.

Type of Ward Other: This refers to general; surgical; orthopaedic or any other ward which may contain elderly patients.

Name and Status of respondent: This refers to name of person completing form and whether they are Medical Staff/ Nursing Staff/Social Worker/ Occupational Therapist etc.

Date of assessment: This refers to date form is completed.

Notes: This refers to any additional, relevant or useful, information.

Areas Measured

The areas measured use the concept of **the interval** (independent, long, short, critical), which is the time during which an individual can cope without help or attention. The person who completes the form is being asked to make an assessment of how frequently help is needed. Use of aids does not count as help. Drugs are treated in the same way. If a problem is controlled by drugs, then it is not rated as a current problem.

Ratings

Ratings are based on the level of help or monitoring the person needs (not on what they actually receive). This is regardless of whether the dependency is brought about by physical or mental incapacity, or both. If there are problems which occur in more than one category, the highest (most severe) rating should be chosen. All ratings are based on the current situation at the time of the assessment.

Physical Mobility

This refers to the ability to move around, not ability to find one's way about. The ability to find one's way about is covered in "behaviour". People are likely to need help from anyone at **long intervals** if they have difficulties walking outdoors; they are likely to need help at **critical intervals** if they have problems walking indoors.

Self Care and Continence

This refers to the person's ability to get dressed, washed and use the toilet independently or appropriately. Problems with bathing or dressing tend to be **long interval** (once a day) or **short interval** (more than once a day). Where a person is incontinent, the question to be asked is whether it is possible to help on a plannable basis **(short interval)**, or if the incontinence is unpredictable or very frequent **(critical interval)**.

Need for Domestic Support

This refers to ability to prepare and cook a meal, do light housework or wash and iron clothes. Help from anyone with shopping is usually done at **long intervals** (once a day or less); help from anyone with housework or laundry tends to be **long interval** (once a day or less) but can be **short interval** (more than once a day); help from anyone with meals is usually **short interval** (more than once a day).
The question you should ask is not whether the person *actually does* these things, but whether he/she would be able to do so if required.

Behaviour

This refers to problems caused because of certain actions, or lack of action, by the person. Examples of behaviour which might cause a problem include: wandering, aggression, abuse, self-harming or dangerous behaviour, apathy, excessive dependency or attention seeking.

Support in the community

Informal Care: This refers to main carers such as family, friends or neighbours, not paid services such as home help or district nurse.

Carer Involvement: This refers to length of time carers are personally involved in providing assistance /supervision either with, or on behalf of, the sufferer.

Can Carers Cope: This section refers to the situation of the main carer and refers to two different kinds of problems. **Practical** problems which are likely to affect caring include: the ill health of the carer, threat to employment, competing family commitments, financial difficulties, isolation. **Emotional** problems include: feelings of distress, poor morale,friction between carers.

Patient's Home Address: This refers to the patient's most recent home address, or address to which they will be discharged, if different.

Social Isolation of the Sufferer: This refers to how long the sufferer is at home alone during the day. A day will normally be from morning to evening (7am -10pm).

ACCOMMODATION

Independent Housing: This refers to housing where no supervision/support is given by outside services.

Supported Housing: This refers to housing with warden service or with support of community/residential services.

Residential Care: This refers to Local Authority/Private/Voluntary Sector Nursing Home or Residential Home.
No accommodation currently available: This refers to appropriate accommodation being sought, perhaps after an assessment of patient's capabilities.

MATERIAL RESOURCES OF SUFFERER

House Tenure: This refers to whether sufferer/spouse owns house; rents it; shares another's house (eg. a relative such as a son or daughter).

House Condition: This refers to lack of facilities in the house which make caring difficult:
- eg. inside toilet; hot water, bath/shower, or central heating, or
- whether the house requires a lot of major repairs.

Income: This refers to whether, as well as basic pension/income support, the sufferer:
- receives any special benefits eg. Attendance Allowance, and/or
- receives any private income from savings/investments or occupational pension.

Residential Care

Confidential	Ref:	
Surname:		
First names		
Date of Birth	Age	Sex
Name/Address of residential establishment:		
Tel:		

Type of residential care:

Nursing Home	1
Residential Home	2
Other	3

Formal services

Write in *number of days* in past 4 weeks service has been received by sufferer. If no service received leave blank.

General Practitioner	
District Nurse	
Health Visitor	
Community Psychiatric Nurse	
Social Worker/Care Manager	
Occupational Therapist	
Day Hospital (name):	
Day Centre (name):	
Other, including voluntary groups (specify)	

Name of respondent

Date of assessment

Physical Mobility	
Independent No help needed	1
Long Interval Help needed once a day or less	2
Critical Interval Help needed more than once a day	3
Self Care and Continence	
Independent No help needed	1
Long Interval Help needed once a day or less	2
Short Interval Help needed more than once a day, at regular times	3
Critical Interval Help needed more than once a day, unpredictably or very frequently	4
Night Help needed with personal care at night	N
Need for Domestic Support	
Independent No help needed	1
Long Interval Help needed once a day or less	2
Short Interval Help needed more than once a day	3
Behaviour	
Independent No help needed	1
Long Interval Help/monitoring needed once a day or less	2
Short Interval Help/monitoring needed more than once a day	3
Critical Interval Help needed more than once a day, unpredictably or very frequently	4
Night Help/monitoring needed at night.	N
Financial circumstances of person assessed	
Independently funded	1
Partly subsidised	2
Wholly subsidised	3

Please circle appropriate number or letter in above categories.

Notes

Guidelines For
Dementia Needs Profile
(Residential Care)

The Profile has been designed for use by local Health and Social Work planners to assess the needs of people with Dementia. It is not intended to provide individual assessments but to provide information on levels of need in the population as a whole.

User Guide

The aim of the profile is to identify the needs of the dementia sufferer in relation to physical mobility, self care and continence, domestic support and behaviour, and to indicate at what level help is needed.

The form should be completed by a member of the Residential Care Staff who is familiar with the dementia sufferer. A separate form should be completed for each sufferer being assessed.

The Profile

Reference: This should be left blank for administrative purposes.

Details of **Name, Date of Birth,** etc., refer to the dementia sufferer who is being assessed.

Type of Residential Care

Nursing Home) **Residential Home)**	This refers to Local authority/ Private/Voluntary Sector
Other Residential **Care**	This refers to special arrangements e.g. Very Sheltered Housing

Formal Services

This measures the range and frequency of services being received by the resident. If, for example, a District Nurse has called twice a week over the past month, the number "8" should be entered. If the G.P. has visited once during that time, enter "1". If the resident has attended any Day Centre, Club etc., enter number of visits and the name of the establishment visited. Only services **additional** to those provided by the residential establishment should be recorded.

Name of respondent

This refers to name of care staff completing form.

Date of assessment

This refers to date form is completed.

Areas Measured

The areas measured use the concept of **the interval** (independent, long, short, critical), which is the time during which an individual can cope without help or attention. The person who completes the form is being asked to make an assessment of how frequently help is needed. Use of aids does not count as help. Drugs are treated in the same way. If a problem is controlled by drugs, then it is not rated as a current problem.

Ratings

Ratings are based on the level of help or monitoring the person needs (not on what they actually receive). This is regardless of whether the dependency is brought about by physical or mental incapacity, or both. If there are problems which occur in more than one category, the highest (most severe) rating should be chosen.

All ratings are based on the current situation at the time of the assessment.

Physical Mobility

This refers to the ability to move around, not ability to find one's way about. The ability to find one's way about is covered in "behaviour".

People are likely to need help from anyone at **long intervals** if they have difficulties walking outdoors; they are likely to need help at **critical intervals** if they have problems walking indoors.

Self Care and Continence

This refers to activities such as dressing, washing, bathing or assistance with the toilet. Problems with bathing or dressing tend to be **long interval** (once a day) or **short interval** (more than once a day). Where a person is incontinent, the question to be asked is whether it is possible to help on a plannable basis **(short interval)**, or if the incontinence is unpredictable or very frequent **(critical interval)**.

Need for Domestic Support

This refers to ordinary housework such as shopping, washing and ironing, cleaning and dusting, cooking or making a hot drink. Help from anyone with shopping is usually done at **long intervals** (once a day or less); help from anyone with housework or laundry tends to be **long interval** (once a day or less) but can be **short interval** (more than once a day); help from anyone with meals is usually **short interval** (more than once a day).

The question you should ask is not whether the person *actually does* these things, but whether he/she would be able to do so if required.

Behaviour

This refers to problems caused because of certain actions, or lack of action, by the person. Examples of behaviour which might cause a problem include: wandering, aggression, abuse, self-harming or dangerous behaviour, apathy, excessive dependency or attention seeking.

Financial Circumstances

Independently Funded

This refers to a resident paying the entire cost of the residential care from private means.

Partially Subsidised

This refers to a resident making some contribution to the cost of residential care from private means.

Wholly Subsidised

This refers to a resident who is dependent on benefit to pay for care due to insufficient private means.

Notes

This space is provided for any further information which might be relevant and useful eg. details about any medical condition which might affect sufferer's ability.

Questionnaire for Carers

This questionnaire is intended to identify the needs of people who might have problems of memory or confusion. All information you give is kept totally confidential.

Please give your own name: ______________________________

Your address: ______________________________

____

Your telephone number: ______________________________

Part A: The person you help or care for

Their name is: ______________________________

Their address is: ______________________________

____

A1 What is their date of birth? ______________________

A2 Is the person *(please tick)*

Male ___
Female ___

Part B: Problems with memory or confusion

Please tick for each question.

B1 Does the person you help or care for often forget the names of family or friends seen regularly?

Yes ___
No ___

B2 Do they often often lose track of what is being said in the middle of a conversation? Yes ___ No ___

B3 Do they often get confused about what time of day it is? Yes ___ No ___

B4 Do they often get confused about where they are? Yes ___ No ___

B5 Do they have difficulty working out how to do ordinary everyday tasks? Yes ___ No ___

B6 Do they often have difficulty remembering recent events? Yes ___ No ___

Part C: Medical history

C1 If you have been given a diagnosis or medical reason for the problems that the person you help has with memory or confusion, *please write it here.*

Part D: Help or attention needed

Please tick for each question.

D1 ***Mobility*** *means the physical ability to move around, rise from a chair, etc. There is a question later about problems of wandering or getting lost.*

a) Does the person you help or care for need help with mobility from anyone? Yes ___ No ___

IF NO HELP NEEDED WITH MOBILITY, GO TO QUESTION D2.

b) How often do they need help with mobility from anyone?

Less than once a week ___
Less than once a day ___
Once a day ___
More than once a day ___

D2 ***Personal care*** *means activities such as dressing, washing, bathing,* *assistance with the toilet, taking medicines.*

a) Does the person you help or care for need help with personal care from anyone? Yes ___ No ___

IF NO HELP NEEDED WITH PERSONAL CARE, GO TO QUESTION D3.

b) How often do they need help with personal care from anyone?

Less than once a week ___
Less than once a day ___
Once a day ___
More than once a day at regular times ___
More than once a day at unpredictable times or frequently (more than every 2 hours) ___

c) Do they need help with personal care during the night (eg help to reach the toilet?) Yes ___ No ___

D3 ***Domestic tasks** means ordinary housework such as shopping, washing and ironing, cleaning and dusting, cooking, making a hot drink.*

a) Does the person you help or care for need help from anyone with domestic tasks? Yes ___ No ___

IF NO HELP NEEDED WITH DOMESTIC TASKS, GO TO QUESTION D4

b) How often do they need help with domestic tasks from anyone?

Less than once a week ___
Less than once a day ___
Once a day ___
More than once a day ___

D4 ***Behaviour** means any actions that create a need for assistance or attention. Examples of behaviour that might cause difficulty are wandering, careless use of cigarettes, being awkward, being unco-operative, being over-active, excessive anxiety, physical or verbal aggression.*

a) Does the person you help or care for need help from anyone because of their behaviour? Yes ___ No ___

IF NO HELP NEEDED BECAUSE OF BEHAVIOUR, GO TO PART E.

b) How often do they need help from anyone because of their behaviour?

- Less than once a week ___
- Less than once a day ___
- Once a day ___
- More than once a day at regular times ___
- More than once a day at unpredictable times or frequently (more than every 2 hours) ___

c) Do they need help during the night because of their behaviour?

- Yes ___
- No ___

Part E: Social and material circumstances

Please tick for each question.

E1 For how long during a typical day (7am to 10pm) is the person you help or care for at home alone?

- Less than 5 hours ___
- 5 to 10 hours ___
- More than 10 hours ___

E2 Does the person you help or care for live in a house/flat which...

- They (or their husband/wife) own ___
- They (or their husband/wife) rent ___
- Other (*please describe)* ___

____

E3 Do they live in a sheltered house/flat with a warden?

- Yes ___
- No ___

E4 Does their house/flat have an inside toilet, bath/shower and hot water?

- Yes - all of them ___
- No - lacking at least one ___

E5 Does it have central heating?

- Yes ___
- No ___

E6 Does it need major repair?

- Yes ___
- No ___

E7 Does the person you help or care for get the basic state pension/income support?

- Yes ___
- No ___

E8 Does the person you help or care for get any Social Security benefits because of disability (eg Attendance Allowance)?

Yes ___

No ___

E9 Do they have any private income (eg an occupational pension or income from savings)?

Yes ___
No ___

Part F: Care by yourself, family and friends

These questions are about informal carers - family, friends or neighbours who give help without payment. Please do not include paid services, such as Home Help or District Nurse.

Please tick or write in the answer for each question.

F1 **Including yourself**, how many main **unpaid** helpers or carers are there?

____

F2 **Including yourself**, do any carers live with the person you help or care for?

Yes ___
No ___

F3 For each of up to three main carers, starting with yourself:
(*Do not include paid services such as home help.)*

(please write in)	Yourself	Carer 2	Carer 3
a) What relation are they to the person being helped?			
b) What age are they?			
c) Are they male or female? *(please write M or F)*			

F4 Do these carers themselves have support, for example from other relatives or friends?

Yes ___
No ___

F5 How often, on average, are you, family or friends involved in providing help or care, including supervision?

- Less than once a week ___
- Less than once a day ___
- Once a day ___
- More than once a day at regular times ___
- More than once a day at unpredictable times or frequently (more than every 2 hours) ___

F6 Are you, family or friends involved in providing help (or supervision) at night?

Yes ___
No ___

F7 Are you coping with caring?

Yes ___
No ___

F8 Do you, yourself, have any practical problems as a result of helping or caring?

Yes ___
No ___

F9 Do you find caring upsetting?

Yes ___
No ___

Part G: Services

G1 In the past **year**, has the person you help or care for been in a residential home, nursing home or hospital at any time for a holiday or to give you a break?

- No ___
- Yes - but not as a regular arrangement ___
- Yes - as a regular arrangement ___

G2 On how many days during the past four weeks has the person you help or care for received each of the following services?
(Include services which *you* received to help you continue caring.)

Please write in the number of days on which each service received in past four weeks.

	Number of days in last 4 weeks	If the person you help or care for refuses to have the service, tick this column
General Practitioner (GP)	_______	____
District Nurse	_______	____
Health Visitor	_______	____
Community Psychiatric Nurse	_______	____
Continence Service	_______	____
Social Worker/Care Manager	_______	____
Occupational Therapist	_______	____
Home Help/Social Care Officer	_______	____
Meals on Wheels	_______	____
Laundry Service	_______	____
Night Sitter	_______	____
Day Sitter (eg Crossroads)	_______	____
Day Hospital *(please give name)*	_______	____
Day Centre *(please give name)*	_______	____
Lunch Club	_______	____
Carer's Group	_______	____
Other services *Please write in service*	_______________	______
and number of days	_______________	______
received in past 4 weeks	_______________	______

[Final page:] Please use this page if you want to give any further information or add any comments about the person you help or care for, the services they (and you) get, and the help and care you give.

Thank you very much for your help.

Please return the completed questionnaire in the stamped addressed envelope provided.